HANDBOO

Handbook For Care

Practical Guidelines
for Care Assistants,
Nursing Auxiliaries, and
all Assistants in Health Care

Muriel Flack
SRN, RCNT

recently Clinical Teacher and In-Service Training Sister, The Churchill Hospital, Oxford

– and –

Margaret Johnston
RGN, RCNT, DipN (Lond.)

Clinical Teacher, The Oxford School of Nursing

BEACONSFIELD PUBLISHERS LTD
Beaconsfield, Bucks, England

To Eric and Ronald

First published in 1986

British Library Cataloguing in Publication Data
Flack, Muriel
   Handbook for care: practical guidelines for
   care assistants, nursing auxiliaries and all
   assistants in health care.
   1. Medical assistants
   I. Title   II. Johnston, Margaret
   610.69'53   R728.8

   ISBN 0-906584-13-2

Phototypeset by Prima Graphics, Camberley, Surrey
in 10 on 12 point Times.
Printed in Great Britain at the University Press, Oxford.

Preface

The successful delivery of health care is a complex business. At its best, a wide variety of skills and resources are brought to bear on an individual patient's needs, so that health may be restored and maintained as fully and as speedily as possible in the circumstances. Each member of the caring team plays a part in this, and in doing so each one depends heavily on the contributions of the other. Care assistants, sometimes referred to as nursing auxiliaries or nursing assistants, form one of the links in this interdependent chain. Their role differs from that of their nursing colleagues in that they have no recognised, formal teaching.

A care assistant does not carry out patient assessment, nor does she prescribe nursing care. Her role is to *assist* qualified staff as well as nurses who are undergoing a statutory training. She needs to understand clearly the limits of her responsibilities, she is bound by the same obligations of confidentiality as the rest of the team and she must know unerringly when to seek prior advice or authorisation from qualified staff.

We have written this text to try to offer useable guidelines on all aspects of the job of the care assistant. We hope it will serve as a ready and practical support for those who are still under instruction, and thereafter to be a useful reference source.

We have drawn our chapter titles from the headings of Virginia Henderson's 'Activities of Daily Living', as we do not believe they could be better chosen. Much of the information is summarised into informal checklists, which we hope will make learning and remembering that much easier. The literature references are deliberately brief – restricted to the ones that are likely to be immediately helpful, as well as accessible, to the busy care assistant.

We refer throughout to the care assistant as 'she' and to the patient as 'he', unless the discussion relates specifically to a male or a female person. This is done for simplicity and not to disregard the work of male care assistants, nor to imply that the majority of patients are likely to be male.

We have received much help and would like to acknowledge our indebtedness. When making our initial plans we sought comments on our proposed objectives and detailed structure, and benefited substantially from advice received from Miss Eirlys Rees, Mrs Ruth Manley, Mrs Libby Blackwood, Canon John Barton and Mr Tom Snee. Later on, Mrs Betty Kershaw, Mrs Pauline Hammonds, Mrs Dorothy Spencer, Mrs Marion Buckley and Dr Muir Gray all worked through a full first draft of the manuscript. We are grateful to them for their informed and detailed comments, which we took into close account when preparing the final version for publication. There were many occasions when our task was made easier by the support of colleagues in the Oxfordshire Health Authority, and we would notably like to express our appreciation to Mr Malcolm Ross, as well as to Mr John Wilcox, who lent us his typewriter when ours broke. We would also like to thank our publisher Mr John Churchill for his help and enthusiasm, Clare Little and Angela Harris of Oxford Illustrators for the quality of the illustrations, and our families for their support and patience over a longer time than any of them had at first imagined.

M.H.F., H.M.J.

Contents

Contents

N.B. Blank pages have been left at intervals in this book. The reader may find it helpful to use these to record local information of relevance to her or his work, as well as details of local policies which differ from the ones we describe here.

Chapter 1

The Role of the Care Assistant

We hope that the guidelines in this book will be helpful to care assistants working either in general hospitals or in the community on day or night duty. Working with patients and all grades of staff in a multidisciplinary environment should be a rewarding experience and one that offers a constant challenge to your awareness of patients' needs.

This book is not intended to replace in-service training and supervision. It is designed to serve as a reference source, enabling you to understand patients' needs more fully and to be more aware of the aspects of health and safety for patients and staff in the work environment. Depending on your employer's specific requirements you should be able to carry out those procedures delegated to you correctly and safely.

THE ROLE OF THE CARE ASSISTANT/ NURSING AUXILIARY

'Auxiliary' is defined as 'a person that gives help'. The role of the care assistant is to 'help' or 'assist' members of the nursing team to fulfil their role more effectively. As a care assistant you are not a nurse. You do not have the legal obligations and responsibilities to the patient which the nurse has. Nevertheless, if you attempt to carry out any aspect of care which is not part of your job description you will be responsible if the patient suffers as a result. By definition, you do not have the necessary training to prescribe nursing care, and it is the responsibility of the qualified nurse whom you are 'assisting' to ensure that your workload never endangers safe standards of nursing practice.

1

A job description defining your role should be given to you on appointment to the post, and it should be strictly adhered to. Other documents which you should be given by the employer are a letter of appointment and a contract of employment. These documents are legal and binding on both the employer and the employee.

When you are appointed you will most probably be asked to attend an induction course. This will enable you to understand your role and gain insight into the various aspects of caring for patients as a member of the team. The course should include the theory and practice of basic nursing care procedures, most of which you will experience in the course of your duties. You will not enter into a statutory training to become a qualified nurse, but are employed to assist qualified nurses as well as nurses undergoing a statutory training.

As a care assistant you must never undertake a nursing procedure unless you have been shown how to do it by a qualified nurse, and this must be carried out at the request and under the supervision of a qualified nurse. As you carry out your important role as a member of the caring team, remember that every patient has been entrusted to the care of the nursing and medical staff. You must always be aware of the limitations of your role as laid down by your employer in the contract of employment given to you on appointment.

Although there is no approved national syllabus for care assistants, some fairly widely circulated documents have been written on guidance for instruction and in-service training. It is now generally accepted by most employing authorities that in-service training is essential, and many of them have implemented instruction and follow-up courses. Your main duties as a care assistant will vary slightly depending on your place of work.

In our view the main duties of the care assistant are as follows:
1) Helping to ensure the comfort of the patient.
2) Helping to prepare food, and feeding the patient as required.
3) The accurate measurement of fluids taken in and excreted by the patient.
4) Giving and removing bedpans, urinals and commodes.
5) Assisting the patient to the toilet as necessary.
6) Helping with the regular turning and movement of the patient.
7) Assisting in maintaining the personal hygiene of the patient by washing and dressing, and the care of pressure areas.
8) Making and tidying beds.

9) Talking to patients and being aware of their individual needs.

10) Answering the telephone, and reporting information accurately.

11) Helping visitors and escorting them to the patient's bedside. Directing enquiries to the nurse in charge.

12) Assisting with the admission of patients to hospital.

13) Assisting members of the ward team to keep the ward and annexes tidy.

In some areas you may also be taught to do the following:

14) Take and record temperature, pulse and respiration rate (but see page 30).

15) Test urine as part of a routine procedure (but see page 68).

UNIFORM AND TOOLS OF THE TRADE

On appointment you will normally be provided with a uniform and an explanation on how to wear and launder it correctly. You will find the following additional items useful, although you may be expected to supply them yourself:

Cardigan
You may be asked to get one of a particular colour to wear when you have mealbreaks, but it is never worn when attending to a patient.

Dictionary
A small nursing dictionary will be useful.

Hairgrips
If your hair is long you will be required to wear it up, off the shoulders. You may be asked to wear a cap and in this case will need hairgrips to secure it.

Handcream
Many care assistants carry a small container of handcream to keep hands supple.

Nail file
This may be useful for filing patients' nails.

Notebook
Always carry a small notebook which will fit into your pocket so that you can write down necessary information. Never leave the notebook lying around for anyone to read, and avoid writing confidential

information in such a way that the identity of the person in question is exposed.

Pens
You will be expected to provide a red and a blue or black ballpoint pen.

Scissors
A pair of pocket-size scissors is essential.

Shoes
Ideally two pairs of comfortable shoes should be bought. The type you will be asked to wear will be lace-up, low-heeled and with a quiet tread.

Tights/stockings
These are not provided by your employer even though a particular colour may be specified.

Torch
Necessary on night duty and sometimes also very useful on day duty.

Watch with a 'sweep' second hand
This will prove extremely useful, as the exact timing of many observations is important. (In practice, we find a sweep hand preferable to a digital face.)

THE NURSING PROCESS

This is a systematic approach used by qualified staff to assess patients' problems and plan nursing care accordingly. You will help to carry out the care, which will be constantly evaluated by the nursing staff and altered as necessary.

In her book *Basic Principles of Nursing Care*, Virginia Henderson has described the basic needs of the human being as a person, and the chapter headings of our present book have been based on her approach to individualised care. A problem-solving approach is used, and we believe it will help you to make a valuable contribution to patient care. As mentioned above, before carrying out care for a patient, his condition has to be assessed and a plan of action made. You will be expected to help give basic physical care and undertake associated routine tasks, such as bedmaking, bathing and feeding. You will not be responsible for initiating this, but should evaluate the care which you give to the patient and think of ways of improving it.

Never become possessive of individual patients or specific duties. Your aim must be to help foster a happy working environment, to the great benefit of the patient. A cheerful and kindly manner, loyalty to colleagues and pride in your work are all important achievements. You need to develop an enquiring mind and must have the courage to seek guidance when unsure.

You may sometimes extend your role slightly, depending on the area of work. Before you accept this suggestion, be sure that you are happy with the idea. The extension must be clearly defined, and proper training must be given by the qualified nurse in charge of the area. If you move your job to another area you might not necessarily be allowed to carry on performing these extra tasks. If, after being in post for some time you still feel that you are not being 'stretched' enough, and have the necessary ability, you may wish to consider further formal training. In the first instance you could ask your employer whether you would be considered a suitable candidate to apply for nurse training.

Nurse training courses which are available include the following:

General nursing. This is usually a three-year course leading to qualification as a Registered General Nurse (previously known in England and Wales as State Registered Nurse).

Mental illness nursing. This is a three-year course leading to qualification as a Registered Mental Nurse.

Mental handicap nursing. This is a three-year course leading to qualification as a Registered Nurse for the Mentally Handicapped.

Enrolled Nurse. Training on a practical basis in general, mental illness and mental handicap nursing, and work is assessed over a two-year period for the qualification.

Registered Sick Children's Nurse. This is usually a three-year course. Training can be combined with that for the RGN. The combined course for both qualifications lasts three years and eight months.

Other nurse training schemes are in operation and you can find out more by taking the following action:

1) Write for an appointment to see the Personnel Officer (Nursing) in charge of recruitment at your local general hospital, hospital for the mentally ill, or hospital for the mentally handicapped.

2) Contact a job centre or employment office of the Employment Service Agency or an officer of the Careers Service.

3) Write to the District Nursing Officer at your District Health Authority.

4) Contact the English National Board Careers Advisory Centre, 26 Margaret Street, London W1N 7LB. Tel: 01-631 0979.

There are some major common elements in the care assistant's work which we will now consider.

MAINTAINING THE PATIENT'S INDEPENDENCE AND INDIVIDUALITY

Patients are people. They are also individuals with natural desires and instincts, just like you. It is good to remember this when you are helping to care for them, and try to imagine yourself or a member of your family as the patient. If you have been a patient yourself you will appreciate the point more readily. Patients in hospital, afraid and anxious, have been heard to say that they are not individuals, and feel depersonalised and just a number on a list. This is very sad. Be sure in your day-to-day work that such accusations are not made against you.

It is hoped the following Do's and Don'ts will prove useful. (As you gain experience you will realise that there are many more.)

Do explain to the patient what you are going to do, and why.

Do remember that the patient must be agreeable to any care procedure. If the patient is unconscious, or unable to understand fully what is happening to him due to brain damage or mental incapacity, permission for overall care is usually requested from the relatives by the doctors and qualified nurses. To perform any procedure without the consent of the patient or relatives could be interpreted as assault, which is a criminal act and punishable by law.

Do remember that privacy for the patient is essential. This is shown, as one example, by using curtains or screens, or closing doors in toilet and bath areas when care is given.

Do make sure you know the correct channels of communication between yourself and the person in charge. Never attempt to do anything for a patient until these are clear in your mind.

Do find out from the patient exactly what he is able to perform for himself.

Don't take his independence away from him, for example by automatically moving his position in bed or in a chair, adjusting his pillows, or washing and dressing him. It must be said that some patients tend to think that everything will be done for them when they are ill. This very much depends on the type or severity of the illness. The type of medical treatment will be recommended and prescribed by the doctor in charge of the patient, and the nursing care will be prescribed by qualified nurses.

Don't forget that on being discharged home the patient will need to be as mobile as possible to enable him to lead a normal life again. Patients cared for at home do not always have help or assistance readily available, so *all* patients should be encouraged to do as much as possible for themselves as soon as possible (always bearing in mind the doctor's orders).

Don't get into the bad habit of saying to yourself, 'I'll do this and that for him because I'll do it quicker'. This may be true, but you may also be depriving the patient of his independence and individuality.

CARE OF THE ELDERLY

It is a well-established fact that the proportion of people aged 75 and over in our society is continuing to increase.

A very large number of elderly people live on their own and are quite capable and happy to do so. About one-third of the elderly have no relatives living nearby and many are on their own for as much as twenty-two hours a day. A neighbour or relative may call daily or every other day, but medical and nursing services provide only a minute portion of whatever help they receive. Disproportionately few elderly people who live alone have telephones.

Help may well be needed, but many elderly people resent outside interference from 'do-gooders' or 'nosey neighbours' and become resentful of suggestions or offers of help from anyone. This can easily result in needless loneliness and an unawareness of the type of help which is available and which would not infringe on their personal freedom. Some of the elderly also have a dread of being taken away to a 'home' or 'workhouse' and they do not want charity.

All adults living in their own home, whether rented or privately owned, have the right to refuse entry to anyone. The general practitioner or community nursing sister cannot enter an individual person's home unless invited to do so. When a request is made to the general practitioner by that person for him to visit the house it is understood that the visit is by invitation. Having said that, the general practitioner is still expected to knock on the door before going into the home, and this is also true for the community nursing sister, health visitor, care assistant or any member of the caring team. If this formality is not adhered to, it could be interpreted as unlawful entry, which is a criminal offence and punishable by law.

Relatives and neighbours may well become anxious if a person living alone appears to be behaving in an eccentric way. This might take the form of wearing clothes unsuitable for the season, for instance a heavy winter coat, woollen hat, gloves, scarf or boots during the summer, or conversely a cotton shirt and trousers or dress and no shoes in the winter. Other examples which cause concern are obvious weight loss, irregular delivery of milk or milk delivered but left on the doorstep, curtains closed day and night, electric light on day and night, dustbins full to overflowing, domestic animals either neglected, noisy or smelly and causing a nuisance or health hazard. Because of genuine concern for the well-being of the person it is not unusual for this information to be related to the Health Centre staff, or minister of religion.

As already explained, unless the person in question asks for a visit there is very little that can be done, and indeed there may be no need for outside interference. The general practitioner may ask the health visitor to call, depending on the area, although the same principles apply to her – unless the elderly person invites her into his home she cannot enter. It must be said that not all elderly people behave in an unfriendly manner. All things being equal, after introducing herself and giving the person an idea of what her job is, she will be asked in and offered a cup of tea.

Health visitors are qualified nurses and are members of the Primary Care Team. One of their responsibilities is to communicate with and visit anyone over retirement age. Usually the health visitor works with a group of general practitioners at a health centre and is in regular communication with them and the community nursing sisters who also work with general practitioners. If the health visitor wishes to convey details to the GP about an elderly person she will do so, provided she has the patient's permission.

The following examples are ways in which an elderly person may be offered help, but again it must be emphasised that this help does not have to be accepted.

1) The *good neighbour 'Fish' scheme*. Neighbours provide facilities for shopping, and for taking people to the dentist, optician, doctor's surgery or hairdresser, meeting others in the neighbourhood maybe for tea, card games or to socialise generally. If necessary a main meal may occasionally be provided.

2) An *explanation* of what to do if the person is unwell, and whom to contact and how.

3) The *general practitioner* may visit and assess the medical need and prescribe care accordingly. He may suggest the help of:

4) The *community nursing sister*. She may visit and assess nursing and social needs, which could include contact and ongoing visits by herself, or

5) A *chiropodist*, if the person has problems such as painful corns, hard skin or ingrowing or hard toenails. This may be one of the reasons why the elderly person is unable to manage everyday life – painful feet may prevent him from getting around.

6) The *social worker* may visit the home to explain such things as available financial benefits – for example, a rates rebate or help with heating the home. If the person is deaf and has a telephone, help may also be given by installing an extension loud bell, which can be a great asset. Other general information may include advice about obtaining a hearing aid, or ensuring that a retirement pension is received as a necessary entitlement. The appropriate social worker may also arrange for:

7) An *optician*, who may visit the patient if there are problems with eyesight.

8) The *home help organiser* may visit. She will explain what is available and provide this service if appropriate.

9) The *Women's Voluntary Service organiser* may visit and explain what help she can provide (if necessary) in the area.

10) If the patient is disabled and depending on the type of disability, help may be available from the *local council* in providing ramps to the home, wider doorways for easier access in a wheelchair, or attachments to taps for easy turning on and off.

11) The *Red Cross* may provide, on loan, the use of a commode, foam cushions to help avoid pressure sores, or walking aids.

12) A visit may be arranged by the *domiciliary physiotherapist*, or

13) The *domiciliary occupational therapist*. If required, she can provide help to enable independence in personal hygiene – for example, a seat which can be positioned in the bath, handrails in the toilet or bathroom or both for easier and safer movement from place to place, a rubber suction mat for the bath to avoid slipping, especially when getting in and out of it, or a raised toilet seat for those with stiff or arthritic limbs. Mirrors could be positioned so that the person can be encouraged to see how he looks and take a pride in his appearance. Special kitchen gadgets and aids can be provided, such as rubber non-slip mats to enable the person to do his own preparation of food, and maybe some special cooking utensils with non-slip handles for an easier and safer grip. Advice can be given on the safe positioning of spouts and handles, to avoid burns and scalds.

14) *Cash.* A person may have £3000 in a bank account before being asked to contribute towards payment for help received from support services such as home help.

It must be realised that all elderly people do not require support services. The actual availability of many of the facilities described above also depends very much on the area in which they live. Much depends on the tenacity and persistence of the team to pursue and explore all possible means of help. This may enable the elderly to maintain their independence and individuality for a longer time and to remain in their own homes and surroundings.

Many elderly people are quite content to live their own way of life and do not need to call on medical or nursing services. However, it can be reassuring for them to know what help is available if at any time the need arises. As we have already said, some elderly people consider any type of help as charity, thus infringing on their dignity and self-respect. It should be fully explained to them that the many support services are not funded by charities and that they are entitled to them by right, having paid their contributions to National Insurance during their working life. If they have families of working age they too pay a National Insurance contribution, and part of this contribution is used to finance the support services.

There are many examples of situations where independence and individuality is maintained despite what appears to the outsider to be unsurmountable problems. We would like to give you an example of what we mean, and remember that this situation is by no means unusual.

Living in a village in a rented cottage is a mother aged ninety-eight and her son aged seventy-six. Attached to the cottage is a well-kept garden which provides them with fruit and vegetables. The son does the gardening and takes great pride in this. The cottage does have some modern facilities such as electricity, running cold water and a toilet. A coal fire provides the heat. The son cycles five miles to order the coal and makes it his duty to keep the fire burning. He also does the household shopping. The mother is blind in one eye and has minimum vision in the other, but she does the cooking and helps her son with many of the household chores. She was a patient in hospital a few years ago to have a cataract removed from the partially-sighted eye. She enjoys relating her experiences whilst she was in hospital and saying how kind people were to her, and was delighted to be able to turn a tap on for instant hot water and to have meals cooked for her. She was in hospital for a week and was taken home by her son in a car provided by the hospital voluntary organiser. She was happy to go back to her cottage and usual way of life shared with her son. She enjoys the occasional visitor and always offers them a cup of tea and a piece of (home-made) cake. Her son enjoys gardening, helping around the home, reading the newspaper and occasionally cycling to the nearest betting office. They both rise between 6 a.m. and 7 a.m. and go to bed at 9 p.m. This is the lifestyle they enjoy. If at any time they need help the son knows what to do, but it is doubtful if the mother would. They do not have regular visits from the health visitor or general practitioner.

The Health and Social Services may employ care assistants to work informally in the community where the help needed does not merit the attention of a qualified nurse. The initial assessment of the patient would still have to be made by qualified staff, as would regular further assessments in order to provide any other help required.

Care assistants may be employed to work in the community with patients living in their own home or in a home provided by the local Health and Social Services Department. Usually the people cared for in this type of home are called self-caring. This means they can do most things for themselves but may occasionally require help to dress and wash. Meals are provided and entertainment, holidays and outings may be arranged. The patient (or client as he is sometimes called) can be visited by his general practitioner, who may also advise the community nursing sister to visit and prescribe nursing care. As a care assistant employed in this situation you may find that people have widely varying expectations of what you can be asked to do, and you must be constantly aware of the limitations of your role. You must know who to contact if ever in doubt. It will be helpful to refer to your job description at frequent intervals.

POSITIVE HEALTH

This might be defined as 'healthy living' or the 'good life', even though what you consider an ideal way of life may not be another person's idea of it.

There are basic principles and commonsense attitudes which can be considered as a means to positive health and a feeling of wellbeing. It could prove a useful exercise to consider your own way of life first, then maybe you would feel confident to guide others if and when asked to do so. It will not normally be part of your role to give advice, but as a member of the caring team you will be observed by many who may follow your example. We offer the following suggestions and guidelines:

1) Establish a regular eating pattern and eat well-balanced meals. Maintain an optimum weight.

2) Establish a regular pattern of sleep and rest.

3) Take regular physical exercise – walking or cycling is better than always going by bus or car.

4) Take care of your feet by wearing sensible, comfortable footwear.

5) Maintain a regular bowel and bladder action.

6) Pay regular attention to your personal hygiene.

7) Ensure you have a regular change of clothing. Wear clothing suitable for the prevailing weather conditions.

8) Avoid drinking excessive quantities of alcohol or taking unprescribed drugs.

These may seem old-fashioned guidelines but they have been proved by many generations as good and reasonable ways to positive health. Another old expression is 'take and do everything in moderation and all will be well with you and the world'.

There are also some basic commonsense principles to be observed in and about the home:

1) Provide good lighting. Poor lighting may be harmful to the eyes.

2) Loose, torn or frayed rugs or carpets are dangerous. Remove or repair them immediately, or take them out of use until repairs can be done.

3) Provide adequate heating and ventilation in living and sleeping areas.

4) Ensure domestic appliances are safe and regularly maintained.

5) Check all electrical equipment regularly. Faulty equipment of any kind should be taken out of use until repaired. Large items which are faulty and which cannot be moved should be clearly labelled to warn of the danger.

6) Avoid leaving flexes where they can be tripped over.

7) Provide non-slip surfaces for those unsteady on their feet. Mop up spills immediately and avoid walking on wet floors.

8) Lock up drugs and medicines and keep them out of reach of children.

9) Always make sure the labels on all containers are legible and that you can understand them. Keep household bleaches and disinfectants, weed killer and so on in a safe place where children cannot reach them.

10) Place spouts and handles in such a manner that they do not protrude from cooker tops, increasing the danger of burns and scalds.

11) When relaxing out of doors remember that excessive exposure to the sun is harmful.

PATIENT AND FAMILY

In order to provide better patient care, it is important to know what help is available for the patient when he leaves hospital, as well as the possible problems which may be encountered. Depending on the patient's needs, useful information may be obtained from the medical social worker in hospital, the social services department or the occupational therapist. It is useful for you to be aware of the following points so that you can observe important aspects, and inform the nurse in charge who is responsible for organising the patient's discharge:

- Whether the patient lives alone in a house or flat.
- Whether the accommodation is private, rented or council property.

- Awareness of the patient's financial situation could be helpful if alterations to property are required.
- Does the patient live on the ground floor?
- Does he have a family, relatives or friends living with him or nearby? Do they visit and if so, how frequently?
- Can he manage to go on outings?
- Who does the cooking, laundry, housework and shopping?
- Does he have a large house to clean?
- Does he have a telephone?
- Is the toilet accessible?
- What other services are available to him?
- It is useful to know whether a patient can be easily mobile and whether he can sit, walk, stand, get in a car or use public transport. How far can he walk? Can he cross roads, manage steps, slopes or uneven surfaces?
- Will there be anyone to 'air' the house before the patient is discharged?
- Will there be any food available in the house?
- Is the patient able to get in and out of bed, have a bath or shower easily, propel a wheelchair, adjust brakes, transfer from one area to another or climb stairs?
- Can he turn taps on and off?
- Difficulty in dressing may include fastening buckles, buttons, hooks or zips.
- Does the patient need eating and drinking aids? Can he reach his mouth, cut food or butter bread? Can he fill a kettle, lift saucepans to cooker or oven, make tea or coffee and carry a cup or tray? Can he prepare meat, vegetables, boil, grill, strain, fry, use a trolley, light gas or turn heating on and off? Is it easy for him to open a tin or jar, or use a grater, whisk, mincer or scissors? Can he wash and dry dishes?
- Can the patient wash clothes, hang them on the line and iron them?
- Can he make beds, vacuum, sweep, dust, polish, use matches, light a fire, clean and open windows, fill a hot water bottle, manage rubbish disposal, read meters, turn door knobs, open drawers, open and write letters or handle money?
- Can he answer the telephone? Does he wear a hearing aid or spectacles? Can he thread a needle, wind a watch or clock, control television and radio knobs, do gardening or call for help?

When we are fit, we take all these things for granted and carry them out daily. After an illness, a person may be unable to carry out some of these tasks and may need extra help to enable him to live as fully and independently as possible.

The type of help available for the patient in the community may vary slightly between districts, but the primary aim of community care is to help the patient to maintain his independence (Figure 1.1). This help includes: medical and nursing care, and other helpers such as chiropodists, opthalmologists, hairdressers, speech therapists, domiciliary occupational therapists or home helps. There may be 'meals on wheels', social centres, help from voluntary clubs or societies, warden-controlled flats, flats or houses with various alarm systems, 'Fish' schemes, 'Crossroad' schemes, financial aid, social workers who may

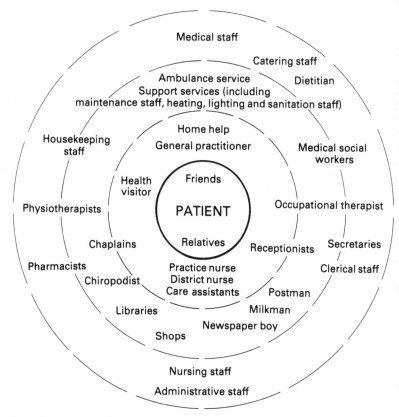

Figure 1.1   *Possible Patient Communication Links.*

organise the loan of practical aids from local authorities, which could include wheelchairs, walking sticks, zimmer frames or crutches. Home improvements could include fitting rails and ramps.

You will find very useful information in the book, *Take Care of Your Elderly Relative* by Gray and McKenzie. It includes aspects such as understanding ageing and growing old, sources of help, answers to some legal questions, personal problems, mental health in old age, practical problems, financial affairs, housing problems and possibilities, carers' problems and what to do when someone dies.

The books we suggest for further reading are those which we feel will help to extend your understanding of patients' needs. They are so comprehensive that we see no benefit in writing additional chapters on these topics.

REFERENCES AND FURTHER READING

Sykes, J. B. (ed.), *The Concise Oxford Dictionary*. Clarendon Press, 1983.

UKCC *Code of Professional Conduct for Nurses, Midwives and Health Visitors*, 1983.

SHHD Health Circular Document, HIC/78, *The Nursing Auxiliary in the National Health Service*. Nursing Research Unit, University of Edinburgh, 1978.

Henderson, V., *Basic Principles of Nursing Care*. Karger, 1970.

Gray, M. and McKenzie, H., *Take Care of Your Elderly Relative*. Allen & Unwin and Beaconsfield Publishers, 1980.

Caring for the Sick (Nursing the ill, the disabled, children and the elderly). Authorised Manual of St. John Ambulance Association and the British Red Cross Society, 1982.

— NOTES —

— NOTES —

Chapter 2

Communication with Others

You will hear a great many terms being used in the course of your daily work, and it will be helpful for you to be familiar with them. We introduce the most useful words as they arise throughout the book under the heading of 'Terminology'.

TERMINOLOGY

Communication – Imparting, exchanging or receiving information.
Empathy – Recognising and entering into another person's feelings.

NORMAL COMMUNICATION

We all communicate in our day-to-day living, and when we care for patients it is important to have an understanding of how this takes place.

Verbal communication is concerned with words, spoken and written. *Non-verbal* communication includes other methods of relaying information, such as facial expressions and eye cont ct, or the movement of the body and hands in touch or gestures. Th expression 'actions speak louder than words' is a useful reminder of the importance of this type of communication. The art of communicating with others embraces all these skills. The patient is the centre of all communication. The 'team' caring for the patients include many people with many different skills to contribute – each can be likened to a small cog in a big wheel, and good communication links are vital (Figure 1.1).

As a care assistant you must be absolutely sure that all communications given to you are fully understood, to enable you to provide safe and comfortable care for the patient. If you are uncertain of any verbal or written communication requesting you to carry out a

17

procedure for a patient, you must say so at once. There is no shame in making this known – it is better to be safe than sorry. Before carrying out a procedure always ask yourself, 'Why am I doing this, what do I hope to achieve after I have done it, and what are the possible dangers for the patient if I do not know how or why I am giving this care?'

We use verbal communication by speaking to the patient or our colleagues. You may be required to transmit information. Eye contact and facial expressions can convey a lot whilst speaking. The use of body contact could be the simple gesture of holding the patient's hand. Wherever appropriate, these communications are received and shared with other groups of the caring team. Patients can feel lonely and afraid of what might happen to them, and nervous at the possibility of having no control of their destiny. Much of this can be alleviated by regular communication with the necessary people and by quickly establishing dependable personal relationships. All members of staff should aim to achieve a pleasant, caring manner and thoughtful attitude, to be good listeners and to impart information to the right people. There will also be written nursing records to keep for each patient. You will not be responsible for writing these or any other reports, but must report facts as accurately as possible to the nurse in charge.

PROBLEMS RELATED TO COMMUNICATION

- Maintaining confidentiality.
- Communication with violent or potentially violent patients.
- Complaints and how they are dealt with.
- The special needs of the blind, deaf or dumb patient.
- Differing ethnic beliefs and cultures.
- The unconscious patient.
- The dying patient.

MAINTAINING CONFIDENTIALITY

Care assistants have access to much confidential information. All National Health Service employees and those working in the private sector are required to sign a contract of employment soon after appointment. The contract usually contains a confidentiality Code of Practice to which the employee agrees to adhere. A breach of this confidentiality could lead to a severe reprimand as well as to the possibility of disciplinary action by the employer, or else the patient might bring legal action against the employee. This is right and proper, to ensure that all patient information is treated in strict confidence. With this in mind, it would be helpful for you to review the large group of people referred to in Figure 1.1 in the possible patient-communication link, and then consider how the patient's confidential information is maintained. This group of staff all have direct patient care as part of their responsibility.

You must familiarise yourself with the recommended code of practice laid down by your employing authority. As a general rule, you should never give a patient's name, diagnosis, prognosis or treatment to anyone other than immediate members of the nursing team. It is unforgivable to discuss these with your friends, family or colleagues, and is considered a breach of the confidentiality code. In the work situation, you must never reveal these details to the patient, to other patients, or to domestic or ancillary staff. Relatives and friends of patients requesting information must be referred to the senior member of the nursing staff, who will then arrange an appointment for the relative (immediate next-of-kin) to speak with the patient's doctor. It will not be necessary for you to talk about the patient's condition.

If a patient starts to give you confidential information regarding a problem, try to stop him and say, 'Perhaps it would be better for you to talk to the nurse in charge as I am not the best person to help you with this problem. I will get her to come and talk to you, if you wish'. You may be placed in a dilemma if the patient insists on giving you confidential information which you have not got the necessary ability or expertise to deal with. A possible solution could be for you to explain these facts to the patient and advise him to speak either to the trained nurse or the doctor. You could do this on the patient's behalf, with his permission.

When answering a telephone, first say, 'Good morning (afternoon), Miss Jones (Mr Smith), care assistant, Ward 12, (i.e. give your surname and place of work), can I help you?' Listen carefully to the person speaking, then ask him to hold the call while you transfer the message to the trained nurse. If necessary, the nurse will speak to the caller or may ask you to give a message on her behalf. A relative or a friend of a patient may also phone to ask for information to be relayed to the patient. You must follow the previous guidelines and inform the trained nurse before relaying the message or information to the person, as it may be considered detrimental to the patient's wellbeing to receive certain information from relatives or friends. Police, newspaper and journal reporters, lawyers or insurance representatives may request patient information. Be firm and do not let them extract information from you. They are to be referred to the hospital administrator.

Patients must be sure that the care and treatment they receive is at all times treated confidentially. This confidentiality also extends to their personal health records, X-rays and laboratory reports.

COMMUNICATION WITH VIOLENT OR POTENTIALLY VIOLENT PATIENTS

Few patients set out to be violent, and there are many possible reasons or causes for a patient becoming violent or potentially violent. This could for example be as a result of head injury, confusion, drugs, excessive alcohol intake or mental handicap. They may seek attention in this way due to a complete inability to cope with the everyday problems of life, or because they feel that no one understands them. A quiet, serene atmosphere and a quietly spoken person can create an initial calmness for the patient. He must be either persuaded to walk if possible to a room away from other patients, or you may be asked to help patients move away from him to avert any possible physical violence and disturbance. The nurse in charge must be informed immediately, and specialist psychiatric advice may subsequently be recommended by the doctor. You may be asked to help remove equipment or clothing if it is likely to harm the patient.

The sooner the reason is known for the violence, the better the staff will be able to give the necessary care. Under no circumstances must the patient be treated with physical or verbal abuse.

DEALING EFFECTIVELY WITH COMPLAINTS

A complaint may be made as a result of dissatisfaction. Remember that people who may be most reasonable and accommodating when they are well might become angry and irritable when they are ill. If a patient complains of anything at all, it must be acted upon as soon as possible. The complaint should be reported to the nurse in charge and ultimately resolved to the patient's satisfaction.

The following complaints are typical examples of what a patient might say to you:
1) 'I asked for a drink ages ago and am still waiting.'

2) 'I'm sick of being the last to have my meal served.'
3) 'Why do I always get a hard boiled egg when I asked for it to be lightly boiled? It's a waste of food. I can't eat hard boiled eggs. They give me indigestion.'
4) 'I'm cold. When are you going to give me some more blankets? I've asked two nurses.'
5) 'I can't see to read. There's no bulb. I've asked the night nurse to do something about it and I'm still waiting.'

These are genuine complaints and a sad indictment against any member of the nursing staff, and an apology must be offered. The complaints above might well be handled in this way:
1) 'I asked for a drink . . .' The patient is given the drink required, the details reported in writing on the appropriate information sheet, and information sought from the patient as to whom he asked for the drink. If the patient is able to give the name of the person responsible, that person should be asked to apologise personally and give a reason for not taking the drink when asked.
2) 'I'm sick of being last to have my meal served.' This should be discussed with the nursing team and also with the housekeeping team responsible for serving the meals. It may be a simple matter to rearrange the routine so that patients can take turns at being served first. An apology should be made and the new arrangement explained.
3) 'Why do I always get a hard boiled egg?' This is a valid complaint. There should be careful planning of the time for cooking a lightly boiled egg (i.e. three to four minutes). After removing the egg from the water the shell should be tapped with a spoon to prevent further cooking. The patient should then be able to eat the egg and enjoy it. The cost of an egg-timer is minimal and it should be a necessary part of the kitchen equipment.
4) 'I'm cold. When are you going to give me more blankets . . .' This complaint must be dealt with as above. If the ward does not have an adequate laundry service, this latter problem must be dealt with by senior nursing staff and possibly also by the hospital administrator. Under certain special circumstances, to overcome the immediate discomfort of the patient being cold, relatives may be asked to provide warmer nightclothes and even blankets. This might be therapeutically good for relatives who are eager to help, but guidance must first be sought from trained staff, since the employing authority should provide adequate bedlinen of the recommended type.

5) 'I can't see to read . . .' What could the night nurse do to reassure the patient? If the hospital policy is to have bulbs replaced by electricians only, then this could be explained to the patient and a request made to the electrician for a bulb replacement. It may be necessary to move the patient's bed.

Some patients may complain vexatiously and unjustly about things generally. Remember to be polite at all times, even when you know you are right. You must remember that the patient may be behaving in this manner because of his illness and anxiety, or because of the particular treatment he is receiving. Suggest to the patient that you should ask the trained nurse to discuss his complaint with him.

Any breakdown in communications causes unnecessary trauma, discomfort and distress to the patient. Complaints can be made not only verbally by patients but also by letter. When a letter of complaint is received, usually by the senior nurse of the hospital or by the administrator, it may be photocopied and a copy given to the person who has been allegedly negligent. All letters are acknowledged – the patient is thanked for having written and is informed that his complaint is being dealt with. Further information may be needed from the patient and the necessary apology will be made.

You must be fully familiar with the complaints procedure currently in operation. Ultimately, formal machinery of this kind can play an important part in ensuring that a more caring and thoughtful approach will be taken by all members of staff.

OBTAINING CONFIDENTIAL INFORMATION NEEDED FOR PATIENT CARE

At home
A patient being nursed at home may be seen initially by the general practitioner or the community nursing sister, either of whom will request and record the necessary details. The community nursing sister will also record nursing details of home care given on the nursing notes kept in the patient's home. This enables continuing communication to be maintained among the nursing staff who are caring for the patient.

In hospital
Information will initially be obtained from the patient, and if necessary, a relative, as soon as may be suitable after admission to a

ward. The responsibility for obtaining information and where it is to be recorded will depend on the area of patient care. The doctor is in charge of the medical care of the patient, and registered nurses will obtain nursing information.

PATIENTS WITH IMPAIRED SENSES

Blind or partially-sighted patients
Blind patients in hospital are particularly vulnerable to stress and anxiety. They are not in a familiar environment and need extra time and care for such things to be explained to them as the geography of the ward and the position of the bed, bedside locker, toilets, dayroom and call-bell.

Arrangements may be made for a relative to stay with the patient until full orientation has been established. This is beneficial to both patient and staff. It is helpful to know the background history of his disability: Was he blind at birth? When did his disability occur? Was it due to accident, infection or eye disease, and are both eyes affected? These details will provide a better understanding of the patient's problems but, again, it will not be your responsibility to obtain them.

Spectacles may be beneficial for partially-sighted patients. It is thoughtless to offer dirty spectacles to a patient. If necessary, clean them.

Communication for the blind patient will be verbal and by touch. A reassuring atmosphere, and evident awareness of his possible anxieties, are essential to promote safe and comfortable care. Provision must be made for such special needs as walking sticks, braille books and clocks. A member of the nursing team should accompany him whenever necessary. It is usual to request his permission for other patients and ward staff to be informed that he is blind, to avoid unnecessary trauma or anxiety.

It must always be remembered that blind patients are individuals and must in no way be spoken to as children. Blindness does not inhibit other factors – more often it increases the sensitivity to smell, touch and hearing. The blind are also more aware of a calm or tense atmosphere. While the patient is in hospital or at home, contact could be made with various societies for the blind if he so wishes. Further details are given in the *Directory of Agencies for the Blind*, which is available in most public libraries.

Deaf patients

Deaf patients in hospital are also particularly vulnerable to stress and anxiety. They are not in a familiar environment and extra time, care and thought must be given to their special needs. Here again it is helpful to know the background history: Was he deaf at birth? When did the deafness occur? Was it a result of a head injury or infection, and are both ears affected? Is the voice production greatly distorted? These details will give a better understanding of the patient's individual problems and enable the nursing staff to offer caring and thoughtful treatment. The information will initially be obtained by the nursing staff from the patient as well as from a relative, if possible, as soon as is convenient after admission to a ward.

Ask if the patient uses a hearing aid. Do the batteries need changing? Does the patient lip-read only or use a deaf aid as well? If he lip-reads only, it is of the utmost importance that you look at him while talking and that you speak clearly, formulating words accurately. Many deaf patients also use sign language, using hands, fingers, face and body. The patient using a deaf aid must always have the instrument with him – should special investigations such as X-rays or laboratory tests be necessary, or surgery, the deaf aid must be there to allow proper understanding of all advance information and instructions, to avoid causing him undue anxiety. The deaf aid must be available during a surgical operation, if the patient is anaesthetised fully, so that when he is recovering from anaesthesia he can communicate with nursing staff.

While the patient is in hospital or being cared for at home, it is useful to know about local societies, clubs and other services for the deaf. It may also be useful to enlist the services of a speech therapist.

The dumb patient

A hospital patient who is dumb will almost certainly be very anxious regarding communication. He will wonder if he will understand and be understood. How will he understand anything at all, and how will two-way communication be possible? An added disability could be deafness. Stop and think how you would feel. What would you do and what would you expect from anyone caring for you if you were a patient? A great deal of understanding, patience, skill and ingenuity is needed by all the nursing and ward team. The patient's particular anxieties and needs must be found out. When it is known by the ward sister that a dumb patient is to be admitted, careful planning and arrangements should be made. His general practitioner and the community nursing sister should be contacted and discussions arranged with them, ideally including the patient, relatives or a friend, or an interpreter if sign language is used. If possible, arrangements should be made for the patient to be accompanied by a relative, friend or interpreter on the ward, and for the necessary accommodation to be provided. This would allay most anxieties for him, and also give reassurance that communications would be correctly and fully understood. If these arrangements are not possible, the medical social worker may be able to assist. She could arrange to meet the patient and plan times for a suitable interpreter to be available. All avenues of communication must be explored on the patient's behalf so that he is not disadvantaged by his disability. He may for example use a word processor at home and be able to bring this to hospital, or while in hospital he could be taught how to use this or other types of aid.

The most common method of communication used between dumb people is sign language. Lip-reading can be another form of communication for the dumb patient. The caring team should have a full understanding and awareness of the patient's needs.

The unconscious patient
You will never be responsible for caring for an unconscious patient, but you may be asked to assist a trained nurse with certain procedures. The unconscious patient is without any of the senses. This means he cannot speak, move, hear, see, taste, smell or respond to touch. As he regains consciousness he will gradually become aware of surroundings and voices, so you must talk to him and explain what you are doing, even though he may be unable to reply. The utmost privacy must be provided when carrying out any procedure for him.

Whenever possible, the patient's relatives and friends are encouraged to stay and talk to the patient, or else just hold his hand. Favourite tapes can sometimes be played, even though the patient is unconscious. You may be asked to provide relatives with comfortable chairs or light refreshments.

COMMUNICATION PROBLEMS ASSOCIATED WITH DEATH AND DYING

The dying patient
Dying, or terminal illness, is the final stage of a fatal disease. Patients who are terminally ill are not necessarily unconscious, and indeed some remain fully conscious until death. The nursing staff will be

aware of the disease which has created the final stage of life and of the patient's and family's understanding of the situation.

Unnecessary confusion can arise for both patient and relatives if members of the caring team answer questions differently. The patient or relatives may ask you questions which you feel you can answer, even though it is not your responsibility to divulge any information. You could explain to them that you are there to assist the qualified nurse who is responsible for the patient, and that you will get her to talk to them. Explain that she is more knowledgeable and can therefore give more accurate information. If necessary, the nurse can make an appointment for the relatives to speak with the doctor.

As far as is both possible and safe, requests are honoured and nursing care is given as required for any patient. As the illness progresses the dying patient is made as comfortable as possible and is nursed either in bed or a chair. Light meals or frequent refreshing fluids are offered. The patient is moved and turned regularly to prevent sores developing, and is helped with personal hygiene in any way that is appropriate.

The total comfort of the patient day and night is essential, and to this end the patient must be as free as possible of pain. It is the responsibility of each member of the caring team to be alert and to report immediately if the patient complains of pain, so that the doctor can prescribe the necessary drugs which the qualified staff will give.

An understanding, polite manner and cheerful approach while caring for the terminally ill patient is absolutely essential, as is regular communication by normal conversation. The dignity of the patient must be maintained and he should be encouraged to be independent for as long as possible. The aim is that he should be nursed in a quiet, serene atmosphere without commotion or undue emotion.

Patients may feel the need for spiritual guidance. If the patient's own vicar, minister or priest is not available, then either the hospital chaplain must be contacted or else there is usually a named local member of a church who is willing to be called. Catholic patients may receive the 'Sacrament of the Sick'. Patients of other cultures will have needs which can be met by visiting ministers of their own religion.

Helping to care for a terminally ill patient is stressful to all the caring team. You may feel anxious and upset when the patient's condition deteriorates – this is by no means unusual. Junior nurses are known to be especially anxious and disturbed by the death of patients. All of us have to try to be aware of the needs of one another. Do not be frightened to discuss your particular needs and anxieties with the nurse in charge. This will help her to give you support so that patient and relatives may have the best possible care.

Many dying patients and their relatives will ask, 'How long have I/has he got to live?' This creates a dilemma for the staff as there is no way of knowing the answer. Insist on being told how you should handle this type of question. The doctor should talk to the patient and relatives, probably in the presence of the qualified nurse.

The dying patient at home

At home, the dying patient's relatives will also need continuous moral support, empathy and understanding. If the relatives give permission, neighbours may be asked to help with shopping, laundry and food preparation. 'Home help' may be available or 'meals on wheels' arranged to relieve the relatives from general home duties during this very stressful time. The community nursing sister (previously known as the district nurse) will be able to arrange these facilities. All requests by the patient must be honoured as far as possible.

Death with dignity

Not all patients who are nursed in hospital or at home recover from their illness. Death may be sudden and unexpected, or expected as a result of a terminal illness, and this is a fact which must be accepted. It is a natural reaction to feel very sad when a patient dies, and if you have had little experience of death you may be anxious about how you will come to terms with the situation. We hope you will feel able to share these anxieties with the qualified nurse.

It is the responsibility of the doctor to certify that a patient has died. The senior nursing staff then ensure that the nursing procedure after death is performed with dignity, decorum and respect. You will not be responsible for this procedure, which is known as 'last offices', but you may be asked to assist. Let the qualified nurse know if you have never seen a dead person before. It might help to ask her if you can look at the body and go away if necessary, and then come back when you feel you can. Perhaps the next time there is a death you may be better able to assist.

In lay terminology this procedure is known as 'laying out' a dead person. Many stories are told of frightening experiences while performing the last offices – most are without substance. The main fear expressed is, 'What is the death rattle?' A simple explanation is that when moving the dead person from side to side to wash him and put on a shroud, or clothing expressly wished by the relatives, a gurgling sound is created. This is due to air being expelled through mucus present in the trachea (windpipe). The procedure may differ slightly according to your place of work, but you will be guided by the qualified nurse. Attention must be paid to the requirements of the dead patient's religion and any special requests made by the relatives.

If relatives are present at the time of death the qualified staff will show them sympathy and understanding. (You may not be able to overcome the urge to cry, and have the embarrassment of red eyes – it is worth remembering that if cold water is splashed on the face vigorously, then red eyes are not so noticeable, because the cheeks will also be red.) Practical help will be offered to a relative living alone. A friend or neighbour could accompany the relative home and perhaps stay for a while. If this is not possible there are other people who can be called upon to help with the practicalities after death, but arranging for this is not part of your role.

The patient's belongings are usually collected by the relatives on the day after death. This is to allow time for the correct procedure whereby all belongings are listed and checked by two people and packed neatly, to cause minimal distress to relatives.

The qualified nurse will inform the community nursing sister that the death has occurred.

If a patient dies at home the relative will automatically have support from the general practitioner and the community nursing sister who will have been caring for the patient, possibly with the help of a care assistant.

DISCHARGE AND TRANSFER OF PATIENTS TO ANOTHER WARD OR HOSPITAL, OR FROM HOSPITAL TO HOME

When a patient is transferred to another ward or hospital, or to his home, you may be asked to help him wash, dress and pack up his belongings neatly, checking to ensure that nothing is left behind. He may have valuables locked in the hospital safe, and the nurse in charge will have arranged previously for these to be delivered to the ward before he leaves. She is responsible for explaining any medication the patient may be required to take with him. She will also instruct him on follow-up appointments and on visiting his general practitioner.

After he has left the ward you may be asked to strip and clean the bed, locker and any equipment which has been used for patient care. The disinfectants used for cleaning will vary from hospital to hospital, and you must find out what solutions you are expected to use and the correct dilution. Most disinfectants used in hospital are phenol-based, and severe burns may result if they are used without adhering to the recommended precautions. Rubber or plastic gloves are normally worn, and a special mop may be used to avoid disinfectant coming in contact with the skin.

Equipment requiring repair should be fixed before being re-used. Your responsibility will be to notify the nurse in charge so that she can complete the necessary requisition forms. The bed will need to be made neatly for the next patient, and clean towels put on the locker.

EVALUATION

Nursing care is constantly evaluated by qualified staff in an effort to improve and give the best possible service to the patient. The care is then modified as necessary.

You should consider the care you gave, the work you did, and how you think you communicated with patients and staff. Think about how you could do better:

- Did patients and staff seem happy with the care you gave? Ask if you are unsure.
- Have you offered patients an opportunity to discuss with qualified staff their worries about their illness and treatment received, or have you kept the information to yourself?
- Were you able to share worries and anxieties with colleagues and communicate effectively with them?
- Did you take time to talk to patients and staff?
- Did you treat confidentially all information given to you?
- Was special consideration given to the blind, deaf or dumb patient?
- Were complaints dealt with promptly using the recommended procedure?
- Was appropriate help given to the dying patient and relatives at the time of death?
- Can you do anything to improve your communications with others?

FURTHER READING

Gray, M. and McKenzie, H., *Take Care of Your Elderly Relative*. Allen & Unwin and Beaconsfield Publishers, 1980.

Chapter 3

Helping the Patient to Breathe Normally

In this chapter we discuss a number of general tasks or topics which are not exclusively related to helping the patient to breathe normally. Amongst them are handwashing, the hospital bed, bed linen, and key points when making beds. This information is essential in the care of a breathless patient and provides the basis for various other tasks described here which are specific to this aspect of care. In addition, we also describe how to record the patient's respiration rate as well as how to take his temperature and record his pulse rate. These two last procedures are almost invariably carried out at the same time as the respiration rate is recorded, and we feel it would not be helpful to separate them. All these topics are displayed in boxes and in a different typographical style. We hope that this will enable each of them to be studied as required, without interfering with the main flow of the chapter.

But note: It is the policy of the Royal College of Nursing that body temperature readings and pulse and respiration rates (T.P.R.) are to be made only by qualified nursing staff or by persons undergoing statutory training, and that these measurements are not to be delegated to unqualified personnel. The reason is that the qualified nurse and the person undergoing statutory training are trained to recognise variations which may be of vital significance for the patient's treatment and care. Care assistants are not taught this particular skill, and the consequence of any error could potentially be serious. Allegations of professional negligence may also arise. However, in an imperfect and understaffed world you may in fact be asked to record these measurements for a patient, even though you will not be asked to interpret the results. In this case, ensure that the qualified nurse knows of the RCN's position in this matter and then proceed as instructed by her or him.

TERMINOLOGY

Asphyxia – Suffocation.

Axilla – Armpit.

Cardiac arrest – Sudden stopping of heart beat.

Cross-infection – Spread of infection from one person to another.

Celsius (°C) – Unit of heat.

Cyanosis – Dark bluish discolouration of the skin, especially lips, fingers and toes.

Diaphragm – Muscular partition between the abdomen and thorax.

Dyspnoea – Difficulty in breathing.

Expectorate – Cough or spit from lungs.

Haemoptysis – Bright red frothy blood coughed from the lungs.

Inhalation – An agent to be breathed in as a vapour.

Mucus – White sticky secretion.

Oral – By mouth.

Productive cough – Cough which brings forth sputum or mucus.

Pulse – Rate of the heartbeat which can be felt when an artery near the surface of the skin is pressed lightly against an underlying bone.

Purulent – Pus-like.

Respiration – Breathing. Single inhalation and expiration.

Self-registering clinical thermometer – Thermometer which records the body temperature even when removed from the patient.

Sputum – Mucus or phlegm expectorated from the lungs, i.e. not spit (saliva).

Stridor – Harsh grating sound when breathing.

Tenacious – Sticky.

NORMAL BREATHING

A healthy person enjoying everyday life does not stop to think about his regular habits and functions. Normal breathing is unobtrusive, and people are unaware of this process unless abnormal circumstances force it to their attention.

Breathing is the natural function of inhaling and exhaling air (Figure 3.1, overleaf). This process is known as respiration (inspiration and expiration). During inspiration oxygen is taken in from the atmosphere, and during expiration carbon dioxide is expelled. The action of the heart carries oxygen via the blood to the body, providing energy and keeping the body working properly. Carbon dioxide, the

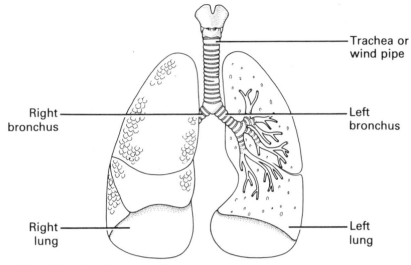

Figure 3.1 *The Respiratory Tract.*

waste product, is removed as part of the same process and is breathed out.

The respiration rate is counted after the cycle of inspiration and expiration is complete; that is, one breath in and one breath out equals one respiration. Respiration can be counted by observing the rise and fall of the chest over a given period of time. The average adult's respiration rate is between 18 and 22 breaths per minute, although the rate is influenced by age (faster in an infant – up to 44 per minute), change of mood and emotion. Respiration increases normally during exercise – the muscles require more oxygen and the heart beats faster to carry oxygen to the tissues, and so the pulse rate will also be increased. The respiration rate decreases normally in rest and sleep. Fear, anxiety, speaking, eating and laughing also cause minor variations.

MAJOR PROBLEMS

PROBLEMS (which must be reported to qualified staff)	DESIRED OUTCOME (for patient)
1) Sore throat	Relief for patient
2) Cough	Patient stops coughing

3) Patient is a smoker and is unable or unwilling to stop or reduce the number of cigarettes smoked	Patient feels better after stopping smoking or reducing the amount smoked
4) Patient produces sputum	Patient gets rid of increased secretions
5) Patient coughs up bright red frothy blood (haemoptysis)	Haemoptysis disappears
6) Nasal congestion (catarrh)	Patient can breathe through nose in normal way
7) Patient is breathless lying down and/or sitting up	Breathlessness is relieved
8) Patient is dyspnoeic – interferes with speaking, eating drinking, mobilising, sleeping and other daily activities	Patient is helped to communicate, is given small, light, nourishing meals frequently, is given peace and quiet to rest between treatment and nursing care
9) Patient has a respiratory infection	Infection clears up
10) Patient has allergies causing breathing problems	Breathing problems disappear
11) Patient's temperature and/or respiration rate increases or decreases unduly	Temperature is normal; breathing is easier.
12) Pain	Relief of pain
13) Change of environment	Patient is welcomed to new surroundings and is allowed to follow own routine, as far as is possible and according to his ability. Unfamiliar routines are carefully explained to him
14) Anxiety	Anxiety is allayed
15) Inadequate ventilation	Well-ventilated environment
16) Cyanosis	Patient feels less tired and is aware of improved colour
17) Patient chokes or stops breathing	Clear airway. Starts breathing

ACTION TO HELP RESOLVE PROBLEMS

It is the responsibility of the qualified nurse to assess and plan the patient's nursing care. Each patient will have individual needs, but many with breathing problems will have needs which are similar. Remember that you will be working under the guidance of a qualified nurse at all times and will be told what is required of you.

1) *Sore throat*
It will not be your responsibility to give prescribed medication, but you may be asked to offer soothing drinks to provide relief.

2) *Cough*
A cough is a sudden noisy expulsion of air from the lungs, caused by temporary irritation of the windpipe, and it could be due to a sore throat. Equally, a sore throat may be caused by constant coughing, which can be very exhausting for the patient. It is nature's way of keeping the respiratory tract clear. The patient becomes distressed and the cough may prevent him from sleeping. A cough may be productive of phlegm or sputum, or it may be dry, and the treatment prescribed will vary accordingly. After an operation the patient may be encouraged to cough to remove excess secretions from the lungs and thus reduce the possibility of infection. A physiotherapist is usually responsible for helping and advising the patient. You may possibly be taught how to encourage the patient to cough, for example by holding his chest with your hands. You should not attempt to do this on your own, but only if instructed to do so by the qualified nurse who is looking after the patient. You should observe and report how often and length of time a cough lasts. A patient may suppress a cough if in pain. A cough may be worse in the morning when the patient awakes. It may be hacking, short, frequent, shallow and feeble, or reflex due to some irritation.

3) *Smoking*
Smoking has been shown beyond doubt to exacerbate illness, as well as irritating the respiratory tract and causing further coughing. There is now overwhelming evidence to show that it is responsible for many medical problems, and the habit is increasingly becoming socially unacceptable. You can set a good example by refraining yourself, and can encourage people to stop smoking or at least drastically reduce the number of cigarettes they smoke. It can also be pointed out that

smoking pollutes the air for others. On the other hand, it must be remembered that a cigarette or pipe may help relieve tension in some long-term, regular smokers.

4) *Sputum production*

Sputum is usually the outcome of coughing and is not produced in a healthy person, unless he is a smoker. The appearance of sputum may cause much distress to the patient, especially if he coughs up blood-stained sputum (haemoptysis), which is usually related to disease. He may be upset by having to spit in front of others, so should be given privacy and provided with a disposable sputum pot and tissues. The pot must be kept covered with a lid when not in use, as it is a potential source of infection. Do not dispose of sputum until you have first asked the qualified staff, as they may wish to check it for quantity, colour and the presence of odour.

5) *Haemoptysis*

This may vary greatly in severity. The patient should be helped into a comfortable position as directed by the nurse in charge, and given a bowl to spit into. The patient's hands and face should be sponged, and a mouthwash offered, when the bout of coughing has stopped. A calm and reassuring manner by the caring team will do much to allay anxiety. If the bed linen becomes soiled it should be changed as soon as possible.

Collection and disposal of sputum specimens

A specimen of sputum for laboratory investigations may be required and the patient will be told by the qualified staff what he is expected to do. If he is unable to produce the specimen at the time, a special container may be left on his locker until such time as he can. You may be with him at the time and be able to assist him. The special container will be clearly labelled with the patient's name, hospital number, ward (if appropriate), nature of the specimen and date. The time is added when the specimen is collected. This is usually in the morning before the patient has had a drink. He will have been instructed to cough and then expectorate into the special container. This must be sputum and not saliva. You could remove the lid for the patient when he is coughing and replace it carefully after the specimen has been collected, taking care to touch only the outside of the container. You must report immediately it has been obtained, because it must be sent to the laboratory as soon as possible.

To avoid embarrassment to the patient when sputum is produced, ensure that his head is turned away from you. This also helps prevent cross-infection from one person to another. He should be offered frequent mouthwashes as appropriate to keep the mouth refreshed.

After handling a sputum container, wash and dry your hands thoroughly before you touch anything else. Ask what is the recommended method of disposal of sputum and containers in your area. This usually involves placing it in a container for incineration in the hospital. It might be more difficult in the community where fewer people now have fires – find out from the qualified staff what you are expected to do in these circumstances.

How to wash hands safely in order to avoid cross-infection

- Fingernails must be short, smooth and clean, no nail varnish worn, and nail-biting avoided. No jewellery other than a smooth wedding ring may be worn.
- Wherever possible, use taps which can be turned on and off with the elbows rather than touching them with dirty hands. In some areas water can be obtained by operating a foot pedal.
- Soap dispensers may be available. Where this is not the case, soap and water is usually adequate. It may be the policy in some parts of the hospital (for example, in operating theatres) to use special solutions from a dispenser. Guidance on this will be given by the nurse in charge.
- Hands should be washed before preparing or handling food (including before eating), after dealing with excreta, before and after collection of specimens, after handling contaminated or infected materials, after each nursing care procedure and before tending to another patient. You should also wash your hands after you have been to the toilet and before leaving the ward or sick room.
- Hands must be scrupulously washed for at least thirty seconds, or as instructed. Take care to wash all areas of the hands.
- Hands must be thoroughly dried after washing. This may be done by hot air or using disposable towels. If these facilities are not available, a clean towel must be used.
- Hand cream may be applied regularly to keep hands soft and supple.

---

6) *Nasal congestion (catarrh)*

Nasal congestion can cause a sore throat and subsequent coughing if the patient is unable to breathe through the nose in the normal way. Treatment will depend on the cause. The patient may be more comfortable sitting upright, in which case extra pillows should be provided. Tissues should be made available, fluids should be offered, and the patient should be allowed to rest.

7) *The patient is breathless lying down and/or sitting up*

The breathless patient is usually most comfortable nursed in the upright position in bed, or sitting in a chair supported by pillows with a table in front to lean on.

You may be asked to help to strip and make the bed, either while the patient is in a chair or in bed if he is too ill to get up.

The hospital bed

There are various ways of making beds but the principles are the same. You will be shown how to make beds in your area soon after appointment. Modern hospital beds have attachments which you may be unfamiliar with – you will be given a demonstration of how they work and should practice the technique yourself on an empty bed (Figure 3.2).

Some beds are of a fixed height while others are adjustable. You should raise the height of an adjustable bed when attending to a patient, to avoid getting backache, but lower it when you have finished to allow the patient to get in and out of bed easily.

The bed should have a firm base or board under the mattress. Mattresses and pillows are usually made of allergy-free substances and have plastic covers which are cleaned with a disinfectant to avoid cross-infection. Torn covers must be replaced. Pillows may be used to support the head, back or limbs.

The various attachments on a hospital bed include:

- A backrest to give extra comfort when the patient is sitting up.
- Brakes (which all hospital beds must have). Faulty brakes must be repaired.
- Cot sides. These may be considered necessary for the patient's safety, although in some areas they are not used as they can be extremely dangerous if the patient tries to climb over them. Some patients however, especially those with an impaired sense of balance, feel more secure with these in position, especially at night. You will not have to decide when to use cot sides, but if they are in use you must ensure they are in position when the patient does not require attention. Cot sides are used frequently on children's wards.
- A trapeze or monkey pole, consisting of a trapeze-like apparatus positioned at the head of the bed to enable the patient to alter position.
- An extension rail at the foot of the bed, on which to place bed linen while making the bed. If it does not have this, one or two chairs can be used.
- Bedcradles. These relieve the weight of the bedclothes and give the patient freedom of movement (Figure 3.3).

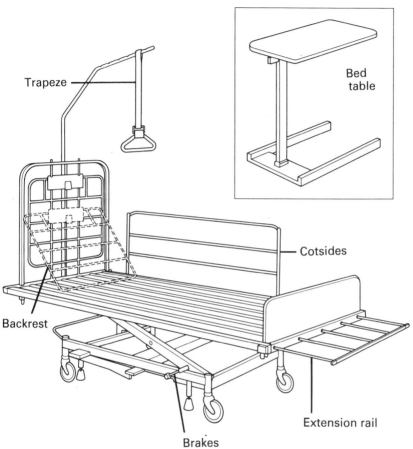

Trapeze

Bed table

Cotsides

Backrest

Extension rail

Brakes

Figure 3.2 *The Hospital Bed with a backrest, cotsides, and a trapeze or monkey pole. Bed Table.*

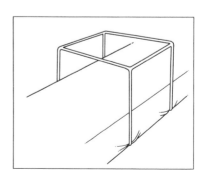

Figure 3.3 *Bedcradle.*

Bed linen

- Sheets should not be torn or creased.
- Drawsheets are not used for all patients, but may be useful for those who are incontinent. A plastic drawsheet is placed over the top of the bottom sheet, approximately one-third of the way down the bed. A cotton drawsheet is placed on top of the plastic and the patient's buttocks lie on top of this. Drawsheets must be changed immediately if they become soiled or damp.
- Duvets are used in some areas, but must be the type recommended by the Department of Health and Social Security.
- Blankets are often made of cotton cellular material which is warm and lightweight. They are easier to launder and do not shrink as readily as woollen ones, which also produce fluff. The number used depends on the patient's needs. If cellular blankets are used, they should be covered with a fire retardant counterpane.

You will be guided by the qualified staff as to how often linen is changed if it is not soiled. All dirty linen is placed directly into a special receptacle called a linen skip. Separate plastic bags, called alginate bags, may be used for heavily soiled or infected linen. These have stitching which dissolves if placed in a special solution, thus enabling linen to be soaked and laundered without handling. Soiled linen is placed directly into these bags, which are sealed and may then be placed in a specially marked linen bag for removal to the laundry.

Key points when making beds

- Save time and footsteps when making beds by preparing clean bed linen on a trolley and bringing the linen skip to the bedside.
- Ensure that the brakes are secure.
- Two people make the bed and work in unison as a team.
- The patient must never be uncovered unnecessarily.
- While stripping and remaking the bed, try to minimise the risk of cross-infection by replacing torn plastic mattress and pillow covers, keep bedclothes off the floor and do not shake bed linen or bang pillows.
- Stand close to the bed to avoid unnecessary strain and backache, keep your back straight and bend your knees. Never stoop over a bed.
- Make a pleat in the centre of the top sheet and blankets at the foot of the bed, to enable freedom of movement for the patient's lower limbs.
- Allow sufficient blanket at the top for double thickness over the patient's chest and shoulders.
- Before leaving the bedside, ensure that the locker and bedside table are positioned correctly.

Making the bed for a breathless patient

Before you start to make an occupied bed, always tell the patient what you are going to do. Unnecessary delay when making any occupied bed will cause the patient to become cold and distressed.

A breathless patient is most comfortable when nursed in a sitting position (Figure 3.4), and cannot tolerate being laid flat. The bed must therefore be made with him in this position, and you will be shown how to do this. The aim is to ensure comfort

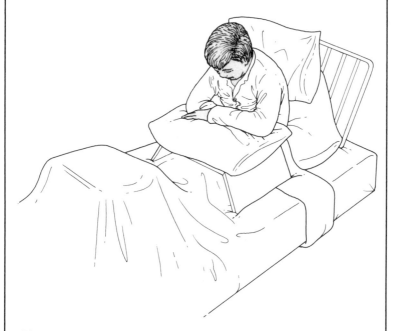

Figure 3.4   *A Breathless Patient in Bed.*

and safety with minimal disturbance in the least possible time. You will also be shown how to change the patient's bottom sheet. A bedcradle may be positioned in the bed to keep the weight of the bedclothes off the patient's lower limbs. If a bedcradle is used, a light cellular blanket or flannelette sheet is placed loosely over the patient for added comfort and to prevent cold limbs. Patients on prolonged bedrest are often nursed sitting on a sheepskin square. These may be natural sheepskin or synthetic material. Synthetic material is usually easily laundered, but natural sheepskin requires specialist cleaning and is not usually washed by the hospital laundry.

The breathless patient sitting upright may feel more comfortable wearing a small bedjacket, cardigan or shawl round the shoulders.

Although the breathless patient is usually nursed in bed sitting upright and supported by pillows, he may be more comfortable sitting in a chair. A bed-table with a pillow to lean on may provide some degree of comfort and relief. Extra effort on the patient's part will increase his breathlessness. You may be asked to help perform tasks which the patient would normally carry out himself, such as washing. He may also need help with eating. Small, easily digested meals will be tolerated best and frequent drinks given, if allowed. Talking may cause distress – you may be able to help by anticipating the patient's needs, wording your conversation so that the patient need only give short replies. Offer a pencil and paper, to save him from having to try to talk.

The patient may be confused due to lack of oxygen, and may require extra attention for his safety. Reassurance must be given by explaining that everything possible is being done to help him. A care assistant who remains calm will inspire confidence.

8) *The patient is short of breath*

Breathlessness may occur on exertion or at rest, in severe cases. If the patient is breathless you may be able to perform tasks for him. As mentioned above, you can help him to communicate and encourage him to eat light, small nourishing meals. It is vital that he is not rushed when eating.

A peaceful environment will help the patient to rest quietly between the treatment and nursing care.

9) *The patient has a respiratory infection*

A patient who has a respiratory infection may perspire excessively, in which case you will be asked to help make him more comfortable by washing him and changing his bed linen. An adequate supply of tissues and a sputum pot must also be provided. You may be asked to offer fluids regularly. Regular mouthwashes should be offered as he may find these refreshing.

10) *The patient has allergies causing breathing problems*

An allergy is an abnormal body tissue reaction to certain substances. Reactions may vary in severity and the patient may know which substances he is allergic to. The irritant may be eaten, inhaled, injected by a syringe or insect bite, or the reaction may occur as a result of direct skin contact.

Patients with breathing disorders may be allergic to the house dust mite or to feather pillows. Flowers and plants may be causes of irritation and they may have to be removed if they are near the patient's bed. Soaps, perfumes and cosmetics used by patients or carers may also create problems.

The reaction which the patient experiences can vary. For example, he may suffer skin rashes, streaming eyes and nose, headache, breathlessness or wheezing. Any reaction or change in the patient's condition must always be reported immediately to the qualified nurse.

11) *The patient's temperature and/or respiration rate increases or decreases unduly*

The patient's respiration rate may have to be counted, and the rhythm between each breath and the character noted. Temperature and pulse rate are usually recorded at the same time. In hospital this is a very important procedure for monitoring the patient's condition and it should not therefore be part of the care assistant's role.

As mentioned on page 30, you may be taught to carry out this procedure, but you will not be responsible for interpreting the results. You must always get someone to check the result when you first do this and at any time subsequently if you are in any doubt whatsoever.

You will be instructed as to how often the temperature, pulse and respiration rate are to be recorded.

The following description is one recommended method for recording T.P.R.

Taking the temperature with a clinical glass thermometer

The temperature is recorded with a self-registering thermometer. Added requirements for recording T.P.R. include a watch with a second-hand, a pen, the patient's chart for recording the result, a spirit swab for wiping the thermometer, and a container for used swabs. The patient must be comfortable when his T.P.R. is taken. He may be resting in bed or sitting in a chair.

Delay the procedure for a quarter of an hour if the patient has had a hot or cold drink, taken exercise or has had a steam inhalation, a bath or a shower, or has been smoking, as any of these may alter the result.

You may be taught how to record the temperature orally or under the axilla. (There are other methods, which you will not be required to carry out.)

Oral
- Read the thermometer and shake the mercury in it down to below 35° Celsius.
- Examine the thermometer for cracks then wipe it free from dust.
- Insert the bulb in the patient's mouth under his tongue.
- Ask him to close his lips and not to talk, suck or bite on the thermometer and if possible to hold it in position. Research has shown that it should be left in the mouth for eight to nine minutes to be sure that the temperature has registered completely.
- Remove the thermometer, read the result, shake the mercury down, wipe the thermometer with a spirit swab and return it to the container.
- Record the result on the T.P.R. chart (Figure 3.5) and show it to the qualified member of staff who asked you to carry out the procedure.

Note: It is not your responsibility to decide whether the temperature is to be taken orally or under the axilla, or the type of thermometer which is to be used.

Axilla
- Wipe the skin under the axilla to ensure that it is dry and free from perspiration, as this could give a false reading.
- Place the thermometer in the axilla. Position the arm carefully so that two skin surfaces are directly in contact with the bulb of the thermometer.
- Hold the thermometer in position. The patient may be able to do this himself.
- Leave it there for nine minutes, remove, read, shake the mercury down, wipe with a spirit swab and return it to its container.
- Leave the patient comfortable.
- Record the result and show the chart to the qualified staff.

Each patient must have his own thermometer, to be stored in a dry container. When the patient is discharged, the thermometer is rinsed in cold water and cleaned as directed by qualified staff. Different hospitals may specify different cleansing solutions and different soaking times.

In some areas a disposable thermometer may be used, either orally or on the patient's forehead. You may also see electronic thermometers in use. Clear instructions should be given to you by the person in charge if you are required to use these.

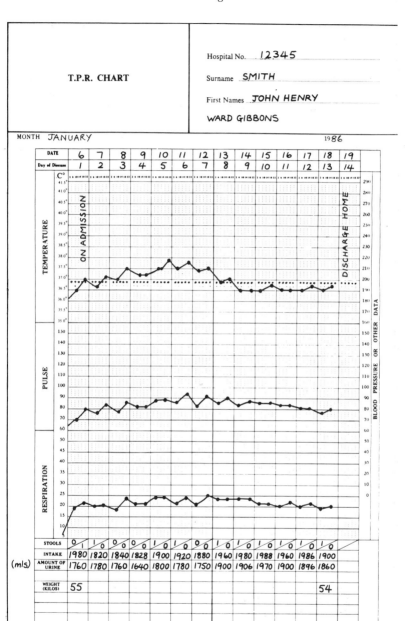

Figure 3.5   *T.P.R. Chart.*

Recording the pulse rate

The pulse is usually counted at the radial artery of the wrist. There are many other sites on the body where an artery (blood vessel) passes over a bone near the surface of the skin and where the pulse rate can also be counted (Figure 3.6). The pulse is counted for one minute.

If required to measure T.P.R., you will be taught by qualified staff how to take and record the rate, rhythm (regularity) and volume (fullness). Record the result on the T.P.R. chart and report back to the appropriate member of the qualified staff.

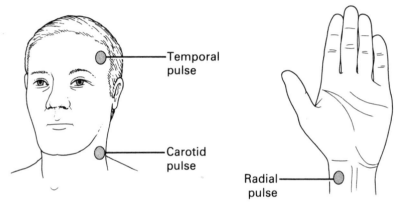

Temporal pulse

Carotid pulse

Radial pulse

Figure 3.6   *Sites for Recording Pulse Rate.*

Recording the respiration rate

This procedure needs to be carried out unobtrusively – the patient's respiration rate may alter if he is aware that you are watching him. The easiest way to do this is to count while the thermometer is still registering, or by continuing to hold the patient's wrist after counting the pulse rate. The rhythm between each respiration should be equal. Any alterations must be reported.

The character of the respirations may vary and any changes need to be reported, e.g. loud, snoring, harsh grating sound (stridor), grunting or wheezing.

Respirations are counted by observing the rise and fall of the chest. As we mentioned earlier, one inspiration and one expiration equals one respiration.

The temperature, pulse and respiration chart should give a clear, accurate and concise picture of the patient's body behaviour, usually over a period of days. In some cases it may need to be recorded for some weeks.

12) *Relief of pain*

Signs of pain may include shallow respirations, slow and difficult movements, restlessness, a quiet, withdrawn manner, or adoption of an abnormal position such as gripping or immobilising painful areas. You should enquire from the patient the type of pain and its duration. Pain may be flitting or constant, its character intense, throbbing or aching. It may be related to eating, drinking, exercise, rest, anxiety or poor posture. Enquire where the pain is and how it is relieved. Does the patient feel nauseated or the need to vomit? **All pain must be reported immediately to qualified staff.**

You may be asked to assist the qualified nurse to move the patient to a more comfortable position. Backache may be relieved when lying rather than sitting.

A patient may ask for milk to relieve his 'indigestion'. You must first seek advice from the qualified staff, as the problem may not in fact be indigestion. Small, frequent meals may be better than large meals and highly spiced foods are best avoided.

13) *Change of environment*

You can do much to welcome patients to their new surroundings and where appropriate to introduce them to other patients. Try to find out the patient's normal lifestyle, so that this can be followed as closely as possible. Unfamiliar routines such as meal times and visiting times should be carefully explained. The qualified nurse will give the patient these details as a matter of routine, but he may forget. Introduce yourself to the patient and find out how he likes to be addressed. Other members of staff will be introduced when the opportunity arises. If the patient is mobile he should be shown the dayroom, toilet and washing facilities. All patients confined to bed must be shown how to operate the bell to summon help. Some patients may not be familiar with the use of earphones for radio or television, and you could explain how these operate.

A change of environment can be very frightening for many patients, especially when they are feeling ill. This may be made worse by the fact that they will probably have to share the area with other patients who are strangers to them. If they are confined to bed, toilet facilities can be offered with no more than minimal privacy, for example, by drawing a curtain between the patient and his neighbour. Some people find it impossible to pass water in the presence of others, even if screened, or in a toilet in a quiet area.

14) *Anxiety*

All patients have anxieties. This is especially true when they are admitted to hospital, because their role in life now changes. The wage earner is not able to function as a breadwinner. The mother of a family will not be able to discharge her customary duties. Independence and freedom are lost, and in addition there may be a loss of faculties – of movement, sensation or speech – as well as problems associated with the change of environment.

You must listen to the patient and try to anticipate his needs. Tell him how to identify different members of staff. Explain the basic routine of the ward.

The patient may have language problems and may not understand some of the 'hospital jargon'. Diagrammatic aids such as are normally available in hospitals may be useful for patients whose mother tongue is not English, as well as interpreters who may be on the hospital site or be members of the patient's family.

Approach the patient with a quiet, calm and confident manner. This will do much to allay his anxiety.

15) *Inadequate ventilation*

Damp, fog, fumes, smoke, domestic or factory dust may all cause air pollution and you will be unable to control these factors.

Smoking. Many hospitals have designated areas for patients to smoke. Visitors should be politely but firmly asked to refrain from smoking in hospital.

Ventilation. Adequate ventilation is essential, but care should be taken when opening windows to avoid creating draughts.

16) *The patient is cyanosed*
The patient will have a dark bluish discolouration of the skin, especially the lips, fingers and toes, due to lack of oxygen. He will become tired easily and will need extra help with daily living activities to avoid overexertion. He will usually be most comfortable nursed sitting upright in bed or suitably supported with pillows in a chair.

17) *The patient chokes or stops breathing*
Choking is an emergency situation. **If the patient is unable to cough and clear the respiratory passages summon help immediately by calling loudly or by ringing the alarm bell.**

The patient stops breathing. **Summon help immediately if you ever suspect that a patient is not breathing.**

OTHER MEDICAL EMERGENCIES

Find out what is expected of you in your area of work should an emergency occur. Summon help immediately if a patient suddenly appears lifeless, does not appear to be breathing, or is pulseless, as every second counts. Qualified nursing staff will decide how you can help – it is not your role to initiate first aid procedures in hospital. You can provide valuable help by clearing away unnecessary equipment, removing extra pillows and helping to lay the patient flat. You may be asked to reassure other patients who could be distressed at witnessing the emergency proceedings.

Make sure you know how to summon help in an emergency. Know where the emergency resuscitation equipment is kept so that you can fetch it for the qualified staff during an emergency.

OXYGEN THERAPY

When oxygen therapy is necessary it will be administered and monitored by qualified staff. It will most commonly be given either from a black cylinder with a white cap (international colour coding) or from a wall attachment if it is piped from a central supply. It is important to remember that there is always an increased fire risk when oxygen is being administered to a patient. The following precautions should always be taken: there should be no smoking or naked flames near oxygen, no mechanical toys and no electric bells or heating pads used.

EVALUATION

All care given to patients should be evaluated regularly by the qualified nurse in charge of the patient, to establish whether the planned nursing care has been successful or needs to be modified. You may be able to evaluate some of the care you have given – for example, did you relieve the patient's discomfort after repositioning him? Ask him if you are unsure. Successful care will have been given if problems have been solved or minimised. If they have not, care will need to be reviewed with the nursing team.

REFERENCE

Nichols, G. A., Ruskin, M. M., Glor, B. A. K. & Kelly, W. H., 'Oral, Axillary and Rectal Temperature Determination and Relationships'. *Nursing Research*, 15(4) 307–310, 1966.

— NOTES —

— NOTES —

Chapter 4

How to Maintain Body Temperature Within a Normal Range

TERMINOLOGY

Bacteria – Micro-organisms which cause disease.

Fever (pyrexia) – Elevation of body temperature above average (i.e. over 37.5°C).

Heat stroke – Affection of the nervous system due to exposure to excessive heat.

Hypothermia – Abnormally low body temperature (less than 35°C).

Metabolism – The process in which living matter is built up and broken down.

Ovulation – Discharge of the egg cell from the ovary.

Space blanket – All-weather blanket made of superinsulating material which reflects and retains up to 80% of body heat.

AVERAGE BODY TEMPERATURE

How the environment changes temperature

The rate of heat loss from the body depends on certain external conditions, such as the temperature of the room or movement of air within it. Excessive heat or cold affects the body's temperature, so that in a hot climate there is a need for air conditioning and in a cold climate a need for central heating and insulation. The coldest time is just before daybreak. People will vary the amount of clothing they wear to suit the prevailing conditions. Clothing should always be dry, as heat will be conducted away from the body if clothing is damp – this is particularly important in the very young and the very old, where control of body temperature is less efficient. A commonly recommended room temperature is 21°C and should not fall below 18°C in the night.

How we maintain a 'normal' temperature
Heat is continually being produced in the body as a by-product of metabolism and this heat is also continually being lost to the surroundings. If we are cold we can take voluntary exercise to 'warm up', put on more clothes, close windows or turn on the heating. The body may also take 'involuntary' exercise in which we shiver and the body hairs stand on end. If we are too hot, we sweat and lose more water and salt. We cease being so active and turn down the heating, move to the shade, open windows, have a cool bath or shower, sip a cool drink or remove some clothing.

Average range of body temperature
You may be asked to measure the temperature orally or under the axilla, as already described in Chapter 3. The average oral reading for the majority of people is within the range 36°C–37.5°C. The axillary reading is 1°C lower than the oral reading. Oral temperature is considered to be the more accurate of these two methods. There are slight daily variations in any person's temperature.

ABNORMAL TEMPERATURE, PULSE AND RESPIRATION RATE DUE TO ILLNESS

Pyrexia
When body temperature increases above the average range, the patient will show signs of fever. The skin is flushed, perspiration increases, and the patient is hot and complains of feeling unwell. The pulse and respiration rate are increased, there is decreased urinary output, loss of appetite and possible mental confusion.

Hypothermia
This occurs when the body temperature drops below 35°C, which can be due to prolonged exposure to cold or a damp environment. The elderly and very young age groups are especially at risk. In the baby the heat regulating centre in the brain is less developed, and in the elderly it is affected by the ageing process, causing the body to lose heat more easily. Old people also feel the cold more readily. Other problems include inadequate heating, clothing, inactivity, or simply eating less well so that body heat production is lowered. The patient may have a waxy look and the face may be swollen. Other signs are pallor and shivering. The patient feels cold to the touch and may also complain of feeling tired.

DESIRED OUTCOME

- To maintain optimum environmental temperature.
- In pyrexia, signs of fever will disappear and the patient will feel cooler.
- In hypothermia, the patient will feel warmer, eat better and be less tired.

REQUIRED ACTION

Pyrexia
- The patient is usually nursed in bed.
- You may be asked to help the qualified nurse remove excess clothing or extra bedclothes from the patient.
- It may be necessary to change the bedlinen.
- Tepid sponging may be refreshing for the patient and may help to reduce the temperature.
- The patient's activities will be limited and he should be allowed to rest.
- Frequent mouthwashes should be offered as these are refreshing, and frequent drinks, if allowed. The qualified nurse will tell you exactly how much to offer and how frequently. If not, you must ask.

Hypothermia
- Prevention – recommend a room temperature of 21°C. If the patient is at home, it may help to use one room of the house to keep warm day and night.
- Clothes – several layers of light, warm material may be best.
- Insulating material as used for space blankets or thermal clothing may be beneficial.
- Avoid a damp atmosphere.

Treatment
It will not be your responsibility to decide how quickly to warm a patient suffering from hypothermia. However, it is useful to know that it is dangerous to heat the patient too rapidly, for example with hot water bottles or radiant heat. The patient is nursed in bed with lightweight blankets. In hospital, a space blanket may be used. A room temperature of 26°C–29°C is desirable. To aid recovery, the patient may be given warm drinks and nourishing food. As his condition improves, he is encouraged to move about.

EVALUATION

Care was successful if:
- Room temperature remained constant at the recommended temperature and there was good ventilation without draughts, making it comfortable for the patient.
- The patient's temperature remained within his normal range.
- The patient was able to eat, and was not hot, cold or tired.

— NOTES —

— NOTES —

Chapter 5

Helping the Patient to Eat and Drink Adequately

TERMINOLOGY

Anorexia – Lack of or loss of appetite for food (not to be confused with the medical condition known as 'anorexia nervosa').

'Build-Up' – A proprietary brand of substitute meal.

'Complan' – A proprietary brand of pre-digested protein powder with other additives.

Constipation – The patient has bowel motions less frequently than is normal for him.

Domiciliary – Refers to a service available in the patient's home.

Fluid balance chart – A twenty-four hour record of fluid balance, i.e. the total intake of fluid less the total amount of fluid lost in urine, vomit or diarrhoea.

Gastric – Pertaining to the stomach.

Nausea – Feeling of the need to vomit.

NORMAL EATING AND DRINKING

Eating and drinking is, or should be, a pleasant social habit as well as a means of maintaining body health and function. Patients in hospital are offered a restricted choice of food, which may well not be what they would have chosen for themselves.

PROBLEMS

- Unfamiliar food – the patient may like or dislike the food.
- Unfamiliar routine with regard to meal times.
- Eating with strangers in a strange ward or dining room.
- Having to eat in bed.
- Anorexia is common when people are ill.

- The patient may have difficulty swallowing.
- He may be unable to chew food. This could be due to poorly-fitting dentures, lack of dentures or sore gums.
- The patient may have a disability which makes him unable to eat without assistance.
- There may be unpleasant or strange 'hospital' odours.
- Some patients may be reluctant to eat because they are not hungry, or because they are afraid they will be in pain after eating.
- The patient may feel nauseated.
- Some patients may have religious beliefs about the timing and choice of food.

DESIRED OUTCOME

On admission, a patient should be informed of the approximate times of meals. The qualified nurse will enquire about religious beliefs concerning food, and deal with other requests from patients such as vegetarians or those on other special diets.

She will also enquire about the patient's likes and dislikes. You can make a valuable contribution by attending to the following points:

- Eliminate as far as possible any unpleasant odours prior to meal times.
- Ensure that food is attractively presented.
- Assist as and when necessary with cutting food and possibly feeding the patient.
- Encourage the patient to eat by offering small amounts of food.
- Where appropriate, encourage the patient to wear his dentures. Check whether these fit well, and notify the qualified staff for further action if he is having trouble with them.

ACTION

The patient must be treated as far as possible as a guest in the hospital. This goes a very long way to helping his recovery. Meal times are one of the highlights of the day and presentation of food is therefore of great importance. The patient may eat at a table or in bed, depending on his ability. A clean tray should be provided with sparkling clean cutlery, condiment containers and crockery, together with a serviette. A small posy of flowers adds a personal touch (Figure 5.1). If a hot meal is being served, the crockery should be pre-warmed, and if the meal is cold, it should be served on cold crockery. The patient is

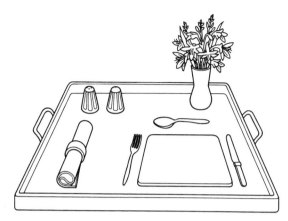

Figure 5.1   *Food Attractively Served.*

usually offered a choice of menu and asked if he requires small, medium or large portions. The individual items of food should be placed neatly on the plate, and if sauce or gravy is offered the patient should be asked whether he wishes it over vegetables and meat. Patients should be encouraged to eat the food prepared for them rather than to eat between meals (Figure 5.2).

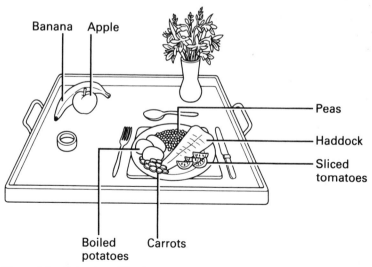

Figure 5.2   *Selection of Food.*

It is usual for the ward sister to request information from all members of the ward team about the patient's eating habits, and she must be told if food is refused. Substitute meals may then be provided. Some ingredients may also be kept in the ward kitchen to make light meals, such as a lightly boiled egg with toast, egg nog, or special products such as Complan or Build-Up. The patient may feel like a small helping of soup, which may be nourishing, although it should not be regarded as a substitute for a main meal. The catering staff will provide the main meals but you may be asked to prepare simple snacks.

Many patients enjoy an *egg nog*, which can be made as follows:

Ingredients   1 large egg
1 teaspoonful of sugar if allowed and desired
1 tumbler of milk (hot or cold)
30 millimetres of hot or cold brandy or sherry if prescribed. (This may be brought in by relatives if authorised by the doctor or it can be obtained on prescription in hospital.)

Method
- Separate the egg yolk from the white.
- Beat the yolk with sugar in a tumbler.
- Gradually stir in the milk, then add the sherry or brandy.
- If a blender is available, put the egg white in and beat until frothy.
- Remove from the blender and add to the top of the milk. If a blender is not available, place the egg white on a flat, clean, greasefree plate.
- Using a knife, beat the egg white until frothy.
- Add this to the top of the milk.
- Place a coloured flexi-straw in the tumbler.
- Place the tumbler on a colourful plate or saucer and take it to the patient on a tray.

All meals must be placed within easy reach of patients. The person serving the meal should ensure that the patient is comfortable and able to help himself. It may be necessary to provide different cutlery and crockery for some patients who are physically handicapped. Non-slip table mats could be provided for the patient who may have the use of one hand only, but could manage adequately to feed himself if the correct equipment and guidance from staff is offered.

Having provided and served the meals, it is equally important that the patient can have his meal in pleasant surroundings. In hospital, patients are encouraged whenever possible to dine at a table, preferably in a dayroom. If these facilities are not available a small table in the ward or room may be shared by others. The tablecloth should always be clean, and a vase of flowers will almost certainly be appreciated.

THE PATIENT WHO IS UNABLE TO FEED HIMSELF
OR WHO REQUIRES ASSISTANCE

The nurse in charge will initially tell you why a patient is unable to feed himself, and specify the extent of assistance required. Thinking about how you would feel if you had to be fed by someone else is a helpful exercise. The patient may well feel humiliated, degraded or useless. Whenever any nursing care procedure is being performed, you will find it useful to imagine yourself as a patient, to ensure that the most thoughtful type of care is given.

The patient must be comfortably supported by pillows whilst being fed (Figure 5.3), having been offered toilet and handwashing facilities prior to the meal.

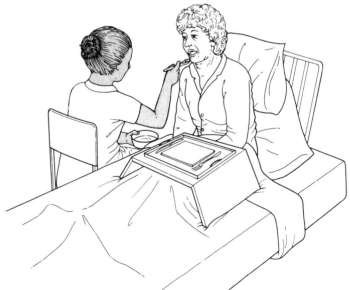

Figure 5.3 *Patient Comfortably Supported.*

You should sit in a comfortable position and in such a way that the patient can see you. There must be an understanding between the patient and yourself as to when he is ready for food, for example a nod or a wink. Ensure that he likes what is being offered and that it is at an acceptable temperature. Before starting to feed him, offer him the choice of a large or small spoon or fork. Protect his clothing and bedlinen with a serviette. Spare serviettes or tissues should be provided to wipe any food or fluid from the mouth. Care must be taken not to hurry the process. Remember that your patient will have difficulty carrying on a conversation while eating, although there is no need for stony silence. Be sensitive as to what might interest him – make general comments while he is eating, such as the beauty of the flowers or the number of 'get well' cards. When he has finished eating, his mouth should be gently wiped with a serviette and then a drink offered, or a mouthwash. He may wish to clean his teeth. After this, he is left in a comfortable position to rest and is given his bell and any other requirements. It is usual to record details of whether the patient ate and enjoyed the full meal. A record may also have to be made on the fluid balance chart. Remember that meal times are a very important part of the patient's day.

Substitute meals may be offered to a patient who is unable to eat an ordinary diet. The qualified nurse will make the decision and guide you.

THE RELUCTANT EATER

Apart from the fact that the patient is not in his usual environment, there are many reasons (other than medical reasons) why he may be reluctant to eat. He may not be at ease sharing a communal dining area with large groups of other people, or may be put off by unfamiliar meal times or different methods of cooking and presentation of food. He may not feel hungry due to lack of fresh air and exercise. A sore mouth or tongue could be contributory factors. Offering small portions of food, well presented, and using gentle persuasion may be the means by which such reluctance to eat may be overcome. The doctor may authorise sherry as an aperitif. Patients in hospital may be constipated due to varying meal times, different methods of cooking, insufficient exercise and fresh air, or just that they systematically avoid the fibre part of the food they are offered. As part of their diet, some patients may also have to be encouraged to drink large amounts of fluid. The qualified staff will instruct you on exactly how much to offer and how frequently. It will be helpful to vary the kind of drinks and to offer hot and cold refreshments for variety, provided that the qualified staff agree with this.

RESTRICTED FLUID INTAKE

In everyday life, nobody stops to think whether he has had sufficient to drink. Usually he drinks when he is thirsty. The natural body process is to absorb the fluid needed and to discard the excess by perspiration, urine or faeces. It may be necessary for some patients to have limited or stipulated amounts of fluid during a twenty-four hour period. This could be necessary for a number of different reasons, for example special laboratory investigations, special diets, gastric complaints, heart or kidney disease, or during the period immediately before and after surgery. The amount to be given will be ordered by the doctor looking after the patient, and it is usual for the daily intake and output of fluid to be recorded on a chart specifically designed for this purpose.

SPECIAL DIETS

There are many reasons why special diets may be required. The doctor may order a reducing diet if it is necessary for the patient to lose weight. The patient may be a vegetarian, or his religion may forbid him to eat certain things. It is important that the correct diet is given to the correct patient.

Whatever the reason for a special diet, you can be a great help to the patient by encouraging him to keep to it. In a hospital situation there are dietitians employed to plan the individual daily requirements and a domiciliary visit can also be arranged. Usually the dietitian visits the patient to discuss special likes and dislikes. She will also discuss with the patient his normal eating habits and what he can afford. There are many special diets, but the more common ones which you are likely to encounter will include diabetic, high fibre, high or low protein, high or low calorie, high or low fat or low salt.

EVALUATION

Helping the patient eat and drink adequately was successful if:
- The patient ate and enjoyed the meals.
- The patient maintained optimum weight (this could involve a loss of weight for some people).
- The patient was given assistance as necessary.
- The patient's special beliefs were taken into consideration.

— NOTES —

— NOTES —

Chapter 6

The Elimination of Body Waste

TERMINOLOGY

Anus – The lower orifice of the alimentary canal.

Aperient or laxative – Medicine to promote bowel evacuation.

Catheter – Tube for passing into the hollow organs of the body such as the bladder.

Defaecation – Act of passing faeces.

Faeces – Excrement from the bowels.

Incontinence – Absence of voluntary control over the passing of urine or faeces. A patient is described as being doubly incontinent if unable to control both functions.

'in situ' – in place.

Nephritis – Inflammation of the kidney.

Sphincter – Ring-like muscle close to a natural opening, e.g. urethral or anal sphincter.

Urethra – The passage through which urine is discharged from the bladder to the exterior of the body.

Urine – Fluid excreted by the kidneys.

Void – Empty.

Vomit – Ejection of stomach contents through the mouth.

NORMAL ELIMINATION

The human body is a fine and intricate piece of machinery, and provided it is regularly maintained will give good service to the owner.

Human beings are creatures of habit, and the body becomes accustomed to the individual habits. If these are good ones they will in general control and maintain good health. These are, typically, eating a varied and balanced diet, drinking sensibly, exercising the body, wearing suitable clothing for the climate and surroundings, sleeping in a comfortable bed with adequate bed-clothes, in peaceful and well-ventilated surroundings, and the elimination of body waste at appropriate times in a suitable place.

The human body has four principal systems by which it expels waste matter. These are via the lungs, the skin, the intestines and the kidneys.

The lungs and skin

Waste is expelled from the lungs in the form of carbon dioxide and water vapour. The skin gets rid of waste by means of invisible perspiration.

The intestines (Figure 6.1)

A certain (unmeasurable) amount of water is lost from the bowels in the act of excretion. Bowel action varies tremendously with each individual – it can range from more than once a day to once a week. It is important that the normal habits of each patient are known and communicated to members of the nursing team. Whatever is eaten will contain some waste material which cannot be digested and absorbed by the body. Much of the bulk in fruits is made up of fibrous material

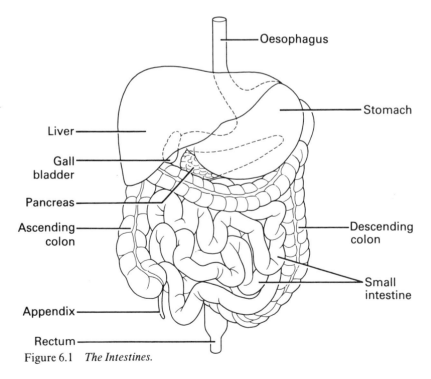

Figure 6.1 *The Intestines.*

known as cellulose. Coarse waste material of this kind is fibre, which serves a useful purpose by stimulating the bowel to contract and push the food mass onwards. The coarse fibres of cellulose act as a gentle irritant to the walls of the intestine, and behave like a natural aperient, so a diet lacking sufficient fibre could cause constipation. The normal appearance of faeces are smooth, well formed, light brown in colour and having a slight odour.

The kidneys and bladder (Figure 6.2)

The function of the kidneys is to secrete urine. They are situated at the back of the abdominal cavity on either side of the lumbar region of the spine. The principal system by which water is normally passed from the body is that which includes the kidneys and the bladder. The average amount of urine passed by an adult in twenty-four hours is approximately 1500 millilitres, or approximately two-thirds of the fluid intake, although the amount will vary under abnormal conditions and in disease. Normally the amount of urine passed is decreased when

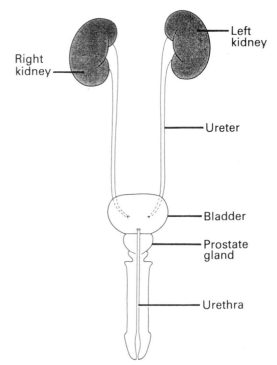

Figure 6.2 *The Male Urinary System.*

there is a decreased fluid intake, as well as in high atmospheric temperatures when the loss via the skin is higher (sweating). It will be increased if the fluid intake is increased or if the temperature is low, in which case the loss via the skin is less.

PROBLEMS

- Increase in urinary output due to illness.
- Decrease in urinary output due to illness.
- Suppression of urine – no urine is excreted by the kidneys.
- Retention of urine – urine is retained in the bladder.
- Ward facilities unfamiliar to the patient inhibit urination or defaecation.
- The patient may feel nauseated or may vomit.
- The patient may be immobile.
- Lack of privacy.
- Incontinence.

DESIRED OUTCOME

- Alleviate nausea and provide adequate fresh air.
- Show the patient toilet facilities on admission, if possible.
- Help with mobility. If the patient has difficulty moving around, the qualified nurse may be able to arrange for him to have a bed near the toilet.
- Provide maximum possible privacy for all patients.
- Relief of bladder discomfort. Medical treatment may be required, but many patients are unable to pass urine in hospital due to anxiety and lack of privacy.
- Continence regained or incontinence dealt with in the best possible way.

ACTION

NAUSEA AND VOMITING

Patients complaining of nausea are usually distressed and alarmed at the very unpleasant sensation, as well as feeling embarrassed. You must be aware of how to help and reassure them under these circumstances. To do this with confidence, you need to have a basic knowledge of the probable causes as well as the specific instructions, investigations and observations which are to be made for the individual patient. This can only be possible by regular communication, both verbally and in writing, with the nursing team. When it is known that a patient is nauseated you should initially advise him to take slow, deep breaths (to allow a greater increase in oxygen consumption), which may dispel the nausea. Offer the patient a receiver with a disposable cover and tissues to wipe the mouth. As soon as possible – that is, when he is reassured and made comfortable – report the details of his nausea to the qualified nurse. She will advise the patient further and also alert the doctor, who may prescribe medication to relieve the problem. A patient complaining of nausea is usually pale, perspiring and restless. When the nausea is relieved he should be encouraged to rest comfortably in bed.

VOMITING

Prolonged vomiting may cause the patient to become dehydrated, due to loss of water and essential body chemicals. If vomiting occurs, try to adopt a calm, quiet manner and reassure him. If dentures are worn they should if possible be taken out beforehand and put into a denture pot. It may be necessary for you to support the patient physically in the position he finds most comfortable while he vomits. You should hold the receiver (vomit bowl) and offer tissues to wipe the mouth. Privacy is essential, so draw the screens or curtains as soon as is convenient. When the vomiting has stopped, leave a clean vomit bowl and remove the dirty one. Offer the patient a mouthwash and toothbrush to clean his teeth and remove stale particles of food.

Patients perspire when vomiting, so as soon as the vomiting ceases the patient should be made comfortable and refreshed by washing his face and hands. It may also be necessary to replace night attire and bedclothes if they have become soiled. Before leaving the bedside, position the bedside locker, the bell and a clean receiver and cover within reach. Ask the patient to alert the nursing staff if vomiting recurs, and then draw the screens or curtains back. You must wash your hands after helping the patient. Report the details to the nurse in charge. She may wish to see the contents of the vomit bowl before it is discarded.

ELIMINATION OF URINE AND FAECES – EQUIPMENT

The following equipment may be used:
- disposable bedpan and plastic shell (Figure 6.3)
- urinals – plastic and disposable (Figure 6.4)
- slipper bedpan (Figure 6.5)

- sani-chair/commode (Figure 6.6)
- urethral catheter (Figure 6.7)

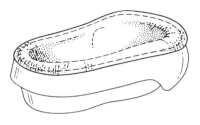

Figure 6.3   *Disposable Bedpan and Plastic Shell.*

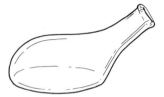

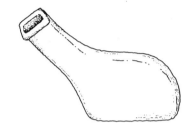

Figure 6.4   *Urinal (plastic or disposable).*

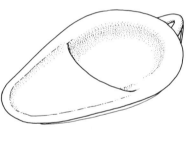

Figure 6.5   *Slipper Bedpan.*

Figure 6.6   *Sani-chair/Commode.*

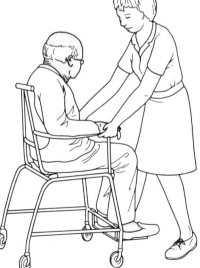

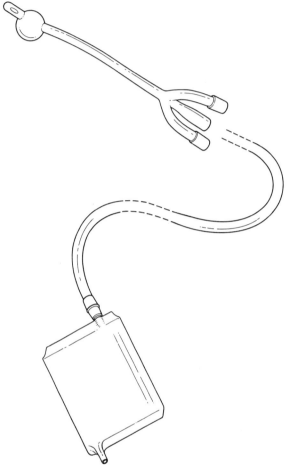

Figure 6.7   *Urethral Catheter.*

URINE TESTING

Urine testing is a nursing responsibility and should not be undertaken by a care assistant. However, we recognise that in many areas care assistants are expected to help with this procedure. It will be the qualified nurse's responsibility to instruct you if you are required to do this. General guidelines only are given here. Never throw away a specimen of urine until told to do so, as the qualified staff may first wish to examine it.

Specimen collection

After admission to the ward, as soon as is reasonably possible, the patient will be requested by qualified nursing staff to produce a specimen of urine. To avoid unnecessary alarm, explain that all patients coming into hospital are asked for a specimen of urine to be tested on the ward as a matter of routine, to eliminate possible kidney infection and diabetes. If a patient is reluctant to provide a specimen you will need to ask a trained nurse to explain why it is necessary.

It may be necessary to test urine four-hourly, daily or weekly. Ideally, urine should be tested within thirty minutes of being passed. You must have clean dry hands before testing urine, and likewise the equipment used and the work surface must be clean.

The patient is given a clean, dry specimen jar labelled with his name, date and time of collection. Female patients should discreetly be asked if they are menstruating and if so, the following explanation and guidance should be given. To avoid blood from the menstrual flow being passed into the urine specimen, the patient is provided with a small cottonwool ball and asked to place it firmly in the entrance to the vagina. The patient is also advised to wash her hands before and after passing the specimen. You may be instructed to observe the colour and appearance of the urine.

Reagents for testing urine are produced by a number of pharmaceutical firms. Without exception, the reagents carry strict rules for use which must be adhered to. Failure to do this will result in the test being incorrect. If you are to be asked to help with this procedure you will be given the necessary detailed guidance by a qualified member of staff.

Density

The density of a liquid depends on the substances in solution. The accepted normal range for the density of urine is between 1010 and 1025. A urinometer is used for this measurement.

The urinometer is a small glass instrument with a graduated stem (Figure 6.8, overleaf). During the test it must be free-floating in the urine, that is, the base of the instrument must not touch the bottom of the specimen container. The density is determined by reading the digits on the instrument at the highest level of the urine.

There are specific charts for recording the result of a urine test and you may be asked to complete these. You must also inform the nurse in charge orally of the result.

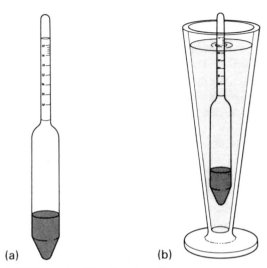

Figure 6.8   *(a) Urinometer, (b) in Specimen Jar.*

Fluid Balance Chart
As a member of the ward team, you may be involved with observing, recording and reporting the amount, type and volume of fluid taken by mouth, the amount of urine passed (measured in millilitres) and measurement of vomit during a twenty-four hour period. This is known as a daily record of body fluid balance and a special chart used for this is commonly referred to as a fluid balance chart (Figure 6.9).

It is extremely important that the measurements are accurate and neatly recorded to enable a clear picture of the body fluid balance to be seen.

Mid-stream specimen of urine
The doctor may request a mid-stream specimen of urine to be obtained for laboratory testing. The qualified nurse normally requests a member of the nursing staff to obtain this type of specimen, but it is known that in some areas a responsible care assistant may be asked to do this. The policy of the Royal College of Nursing is that a mid-stream specimen of urine should be obtained only by qualified nursing staff or a person undergoing statutory training, and that this task is not to be delegated to unqualified personnel. The reason is that the qualified nurse and the person undergoing statutory training are trained in the

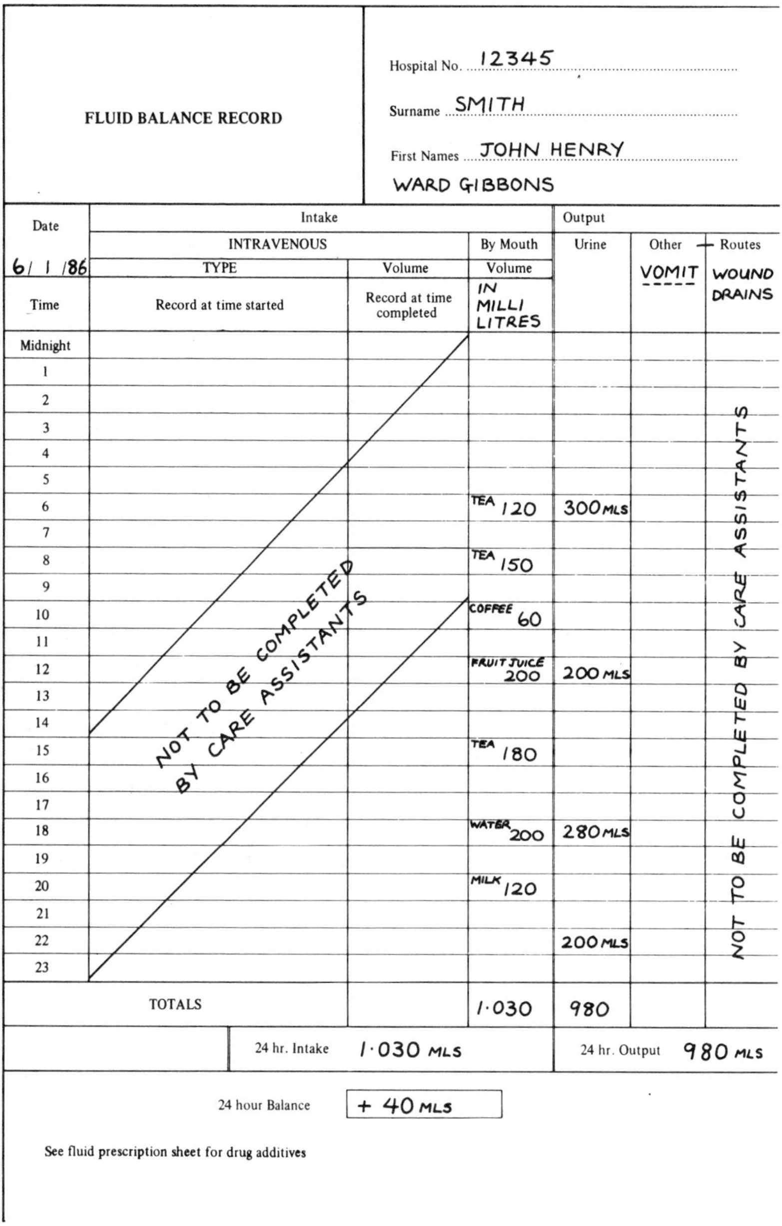

FLUID BALANCE RECORD	Hospital No. ..12345....................................				
	Surname ...SMITH..........................				
	First Names .....JOHN HENRY..................				
	WARD GIBBONS				

Date	Intake				Output		
	INTRAVENOUS			By Mouth	Urine	Other	— Routes
6/ 1 /86	TYPE	Volume		Volume		VOMIT	WOUND
Time	Record at time started	Record at time completed		IN MILLI LITRES		-----	DRAINS
Midnight							
1							
2							
3							
4							
5							
6				TEA 120	300 MLS		
7							
8				TEA 150			
9							
10				COFFEE 60			
11							
12				FRUIT JUICE 200	200 MLS		
13							
14							
15				TEA 180			
16							
17							
18				WATER 200	280 MLS		
19							
20				MILK 120			
21							
22					200 MLS		
23							
	TOTALS			1·030	980		
		24 hr. Intake	1·030 MLS			24 hr. Output	980 MLS

(Diagonal text across intravenous columns: NOT TO BE COMPLETED BY CARE ASSISTANTS)

(Vertical text at right: NOT TO BE COMPLETED BY CARE ASSISTANTS)

24 hour Balance $\boxed{+ 40 \text{ MLS}}$

See fluid prescription sheet for drug additives

Figure 6.9   *Fluid Balance Chart.*

71

necessary technique. A mistake at any point in the procedure could lead to an incorrect report from the pathology laboratory, with potentially harmful implications for the patient.

As with our discussion of the same principle in connection with T.P.R. measurements (page 30), if you are nevertheless asked to obtain a mid-stream specimen of urine, ensure that the qualified nurse knows of the RCN's position in the matter and then proceed as instructed by her or him. It is essential that the patient be given guidance on what a mid-stream specimen means and an explanation of the procedure.

The equipment needed includes:
- Towel, soap and disposable flannel.
- Specimen container.
- Washbowl, bedpan and cover, if the patient is unable to go to the toilet.

To ensure that the urine is not contaminated with mucus or talcum powder, the patient is first asked to wash and dry the vulval/penile area with soapy water before using the toilet, bedpan or commode, depending on which method is suitable for him or her. To procure a mid-stream specimen of urine, the patient is asked to start passing urine into the toilet and then switch to passing urine into the specimen container during the flow, and finally to remove the container and continue to empty the bladder in the toilet, bedpan or commode. There is no specific time lapse between the first and second stage. The first brief flow clears the passage of debris which would otherwise interfere with the test. The specimen container is secured with the lid and then given to you. The patient is then asked to wash his hands. The specimen must be clearly labelled with the patient's name, date, time of collection, ward, hospital and hospital number. A laboratory request form for the investigation is written by the doctor and must accompany the specimen. To enable the bacteriologist to give an accurate report, a mid-stream specimen of urine should be delivered to the laboratory within thirty minutes of being collected. The urine specimen must not be kept in a warm, humid atmosphere or in a domestic refrigerator on the ward.

Twenty-four hour collection of urine for laboratory test
The reason why this specimen is requested could be to determine kidney function, content of urine or to record body fluid balance.

The patient must be told why a twenty-four hour specimen is necessary and whenever possible given the opportunity to participate personally with the procedure. This explanation will be given by the nursing staff and will not be your responsibility, but you may be required to assist in collecting specimens during the 24-hour period.

The equipment needed includes:
- A measuring jug.
- Containers for urine. These will have been obtained from the laboratory. If a container has solution in it when received from the laboratory, do not discard this before adding the urine. The solution will be a necessary part of a specific laboratory test.

The procedure is as follows:

The first specimen of urine passed is measured and recorded, and the time noted. This specimen is then discarded because it is not known how long it has been in the bladder and it is likely to be stale. Subsequently, every urine specimen the patient passes during the next twenty-four hours is measured and poured into the special container, and the time recorded. Twenty-four hours later the final specimen is measured and added to the container. This completes the collection. It is then sent to the laboratory labelled with the patient's name, date, time, ward, hospital and hospital number. It must be accompanied by the laboratory request form signed by the doctor. The time the specimen is sent must also be recorded.

To avoid urine being discarded during the twenty-four hours it is essential that all the nursing staff are informed orally, and a notice should be attached to the patient's bed: '24-hour collection of urine in progress'. The patient should also be told why the notice is attached to the bed. If a specimen is inadvertently discarded during the twenty-four hours, this must be reported to the nurse in charge. The procedure is abandoned and will need to be recommenced at a specified time. The patient must be informed and apologies made, as this could cause needless anxiety and possible delay in treatment, and even a longer stay in hospital, not to mention the extra expense.

SPECIMEN OF FAECES FOR LABORATORY TESTING

The doctor may request a specimen of faeces for laboratory testing to help determine diagnosis. The faeces could be:
- Green, loose and watery.
- Black.
- Clay colour.

- Watery and foul-smelling.
- Hard and dry.
- Accompanied by mucus and blood, or contain foreign bodies such as worms.

The equipment needed for the collection of faeces includes a bedpan and specimen container with a small spoon attached to a screw cap. After defaecation, the bedpan is removed and the patient is given a washbowl, flannel, soap and towel to wash his hands. The bedpan is taken to the sluice or dirty utility room and a specimen of the faeces is spooned into the specimen pot. The faeces may be of different colours and a small sample of each colour should be collected. This is all put in one container. The specimen pot is labelled with the patient's name, ward, hospital, hospital number, time and date, and is then sent to the laboratory with a laboratory request form signed by the doctor. After collecting a specimen of faeces, you must wash and dry your hands and report to the trained nurse that the specimen has been collected.

HELPING THE PATIENT TO URINATE
AND DEFAECATE COMFORTABLY

It is of the utmost importance that patients should have privacy to perform the natural functions of urinating and defaecating. They will have been shown the toilet facilities. Some patients may need help to walk to the toilet or some may be taken in a wheelchair and helped from the chair to sit on the toilet. There may also be a sani-chair on which patients can be transported to the toilet. Patients who are nursed in bed may be allowed to use a commode by the bedside, as it may be less strain than sitting on a bedpan. Those on strict bedrest or who cannot get up, such as those with back injuries or broken limbs for example, may need to use a bedpan or urinal. Imagine how you might personally react if you were a patient, unable to get out of bed, and had to sit on a bedpan to pass urine and defaecate.

When a patient requires a bedpan, you must discreetly assist him, and position him safely and with minimum discomfort. Curtains or screens must be closed before he uses the bedpan. Soft toilet paper should be within reach and a disposable receiver or suitable container supplied in which to place used toilet paper. The patient may need help to wipe and clean soiled areas. Hand-washing facilities must also be provided. A bell must be within reach to enable the patient to call for assistance or for the bedpan to be removed.

After using the bedpan he must be made comfortable by ensuring that the lower sheet is free from creases. If a drawsheet is in use, this also must be crease-free and dry. The patient's night attire should be adjusted and the top sheet, blankets and pillows comfortably arranged. The bedside locker must be placed within easy reach and the patient given books, newspapers or whatever he requires. The bedpan/urinal is covered before removing to the sluice or dirty utility room. The contents of the bedpan may need to be:

- Saved for senior staff to observe.
- Saved for specimens to be sent for laboratory investigation.
- Measured and the volume recorded (urine).
- Saved for routine ward testing (urine and faeces).

It is important that everyone is aware if a specimen is to be obtained for ward or laboratory testing. If no specimens are required, the contents of the bedpan can be discarded. Compressed cardboard bedpans are disposed of in the bedpan machine, and the plastic shell placed in a deep sink with the appropriate disinfectant solution for the required length of time. If the bedpan is not disposable, the contents are discarded. The bedpan is then rinsed and soaked as previously described. You then wash and dry your hands, return to the patient's bedside and draw back the screens. The details are usually recorded and reported.

Using the slipper bedpan

Some patients are unable to use the regular type of bedpan because of an inability to sit up, due to arthritic deformities, spasticity, paralysis, head injuries or brittle bones. For these patients, a slipper bedpan may be useful as it is fairly shallow. Some patients may be able to insert and remove a bedpan themselves, although others will require assistance. This enables them to have a degree of independence. If the patient is unable to cooperate and is very heavy, you must seek the help of a second and maybe a third member of the nursing team, or a relative if the patient is being nursed at home. You will be advised by qualified staff whether use can be made of relatives, and how much help they will be able to give. Before attempting to help with this procedure you must have clear instruction and supervision. This is not something you can learn from a book.

The patient is asked to bend the knees and place the flat of the feet on the bed. This prevents pressure on the heels. The hands are placed flat or fist-like on the bed behind the waist level. You support the patient's lower back with one hand, holding the bedpan in the other. Ask the patient to push up with the flat of the feet and the hands to raise the buttocks off the bed with your help. While the buttocks are raised off the bed you position the bedpan. The patient lowers his bottom to rest on the bedpan. You must remember to bend your knees and to keep as close to the bed and patient as possible. Keep your back straight at all times.

Assisting a male patient to use a urinal
Most male patients will be able to do this themselves, but you may have to assist them to get the pyjama trousers down far enough to insert and position the urinal. Remove it as soon as the patient has finished. Help may be needed to adjust the pyjama trousers. Offer him washing facilities.

Heavy patients or patients who are unable to cooperate
An explanation is given to the patient on how the bedpan will be positioned. Two people are necessary for this procedure, which you must see demonstrated before attempting on your own.

One person stands on either side of the bed. The patient is rolled by first turning the head to one side, and positioning the uppermost arm to the same side. If possible his knees should be bent with the flat of the feet together on the mattress. The knees are turned to the same side as the arm and head. The patient is then rolled to one side, and while one nurse supports the patient the care assistant positions the bedpan. The patient is then rolled gently from his side on to his back with the bedpan in place. The patient is adequately covered with bedclothes and left in privacy to use the bedpan. Before leaving the bedside you must ensure that the bell is within reach for him to call for attention when he has finished. Should the patient be unable to use the bell you must remember to ask him to call for help, and must in any event return to him within a few minutes.

When the bedpan has been used, two people will need to help with its removal, and this is performed in the same manner as when the patient was rolled on to it. You will be expected to clean the genitalia and buttocks if the patient is unable to do this. Perform this procedure after removing the bedpan while the patient is still lying on his side. The sheets are straightened and if soiled or damp, replaced. Night attire is put into place, and the patient is rolled on to his back or side, whichever is appropriate. He is comfortably positioned in bed and the bedclothes neatly arranged. The patient either washes his hands or you do this for him. The covered bedpan is removed from the bedside. You wash your hands and the necessary details are recorded. The second helper, after washing her hands, should draw back the screens, position the bedlocker, and make sure that the patient has his bell and anything else needed.

Patients who are unable to walk or be taken to the toilet, but are able to sit out of bed, may be offered the use of a commode at the bedside. Privacy for the patient must be the same as that given for a patient using a bedpan, and the basic hygiene principles are the same. Commodes must be safe to use, that is, give firm support and have their brakes secured. They must be positioned so that the patient is facing the bed. This enables him to rest his arms on the bed if he wishes to do so.

This is important because if he feels faint while sitting on the commode and is unable to use the bell to call for attention, he will not fall but have the bed for support.

CATHETERS

If a patient is unable to urinate, he may need to have a catheter inserted into the urethra to allow the urine to flow freely out of the bladder. A catheter is a hollow tube made specially for this purpose. The insertion and removal of a catheter is a highly skilled procedure and is to be undertaken only by experienced qualified staff. You will never be asked to carry out this procedure, but you will see many patients with catheters in situ.

The catheter is inserted through the urethra into the bladder, thus enabling the patient to pass urine freely. It is attached to a catheter bag, which can be suspended from a specially designed metal stand on the floor, or on a holder hanging at the bedside. The bag must be sited below the bladder level of the patient so that the urine is able to flow freely.

Depending on the overall nursing care and needs of the individual patient, you should be aware of the importance of scrupulous cleanliness around the area of the catheter and the comfort of the patient at all times. All patients with urinary catheters are at increased risk of infection in the urinary tract. It will depend on local policy as to which grade of staff is responsible for catheter care, and in some circumstances you may be asked to help. Some patients will be able to carry out catheter care themselves. The frequency of this procedure varies, e.g. it may be performed every four hours throughout the day. It is not unusual for male and female patients to be embarrassed when cathether care is carried out. If you showed embarrassment by giggling or blushing this would only embarrass the patient further. Because of this you should always first ask the patient's permission and explain what you are going to do.

NURSING THE AMBULANT PATIENT WITH A CATHETER IN SITU

The ambulant patient (that is, one who is able to walk) must be guided and instructed on how to observe basic hygiene principles while the catheter is in situ. This will be given initially by the qualified staff. He may need help and reassurance.

When he is having a shower, the catheter bag is positioned on the floor by the shower, attached to the stand. The normal washing procedure is then performed, with special care being given to the urethral area by using a soapy flannel for thorough cleansing. After the shower you may be asked to position and secure the catheter to the patient's thigh with an adhesive, such as micropore. This avoids unnecessary pull and movement of the catheter in the urethra and ensures more comfort for the patient. Opinion varies as to whether a patient with a drainage bag should be allowed to take a bath. If he does, it will be your responsibility to clean the bath thoroughly and leave it ready for the next patient.

The patient is assisted back to the dayroom or bed and is asked to call for help if he becomes uncomfortable. The catheter should be arranged in such a way that the patient does not sit on it, and once again the bag and stand should be placed below bladder level to allow free drainage. Kinks in the catheter will stop drainage. The bedclothes should not be tucked in tightly under the mattress but allowed either to hang freely or be folded neatly under.

Some patients prefer to use special 'leg bags' which replace the drainage bag and stand. They are useful if the patient is ambulant, as they are attached round the leg with special straps and can be concealed under the trousers. They need to be emptied more frequently as the capacity is less than that of the drainage bag with stand.

THE PATIENT NURSED IN BED WITH CATHETER IN SITU

If you are asked to help, the information below covers the equipment which will be required and the procedures which will usually be followed.

Equipment
- Washbowl with hot water, soap and flannel (which may be disposable).
- Absorbent towel.
- Adhesive solvent (for removing used adhesive plasters).
- Small bowl (gallipot) and cottonwool balls.
- Adhesive to secure catheter to thigh.
- Drawsheet and plastic sheet (as required).
- Large sheet.
- Scissors to cut adhesive.

Preparation and general procedure
Complete privacy must be observed, so curtains will be drawn and doors and windows closed. The bedclothes are removed neatly and a blanket placed loosely over the patient. Care must be taken that the patient is in a comfortable position.

Procedure for a female patient
The towel is placed under the buttocks. The soapy flannel is used first to thoroughly wash the vulval area, care being taken to ensure that both the labia majora and the labia minora are cleansed of talcum powder and natural secretions (Figure 6.10).

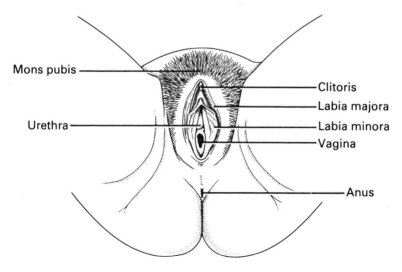

Figure 6.10   *Labia Majora and Labia Minora.*

The labia are separated and the urethra and catheter washed gently. The flannel is rinsed and the area rinsed of soap and dried with the towel on which the patient is sitting. Observe closely whether there is any redness or broken skin or if there is an unpleasant odour. If there is, this must be reported to a senior member of the nursing team.

First gently remove the adhesive tape from the thigh and catheter and discard it into the appropriate container. The catheter length must be washed as far as the connection to the bag. Pour adhesive solvent into the gallipot and moisten the cottonwool ball with solvent. Holding the catheter firmly near the urethral area, to avoid unnecessary pulling and discomfort for the patient, use the cottonwool ball to remove adhesive marks and stickiness. Working away from the urethral area towards the end of the catheter using firm, positive action, continue until all the stickiness has been removed. Using clean, moist wool balls, continue to remove the sticky, adhesive marks from the thigh. The catheter is washed with a soapy flannel and dried, taking care to hold the catheter steadily with one hand and using a washing motion always directed away from the urethra. The thigh is washed with a soapy flannel, rinsed and dried.

A new length of adhesive is cut and placed round the catheter to secure it to the thigh (Figure 6.11). This will prevent the patient sitting on the catheter, which would otherwise stop the flow of urine into the bag. It also allows greater comfort for the patient by avoiding the

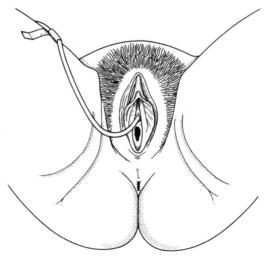

Figure 6.11   *Catheter in situ in a Female Patient.*

weight of urine in the bag pulling down on the urethral area. A useful tip when applying adhesive tape to skin is to fold each sticky end back on itself by about a centimetre to make a tab for easy removal next time. The patient is made comfortable and, if necessary, the bedlinen is replaced with a clean supply, making sure that all creases are removed from the sheets. The top bedclothes are replaced, but not tucked in where the catheter and bag are attached. As already described, the catheter bag and stand must be positioned towards the foot of the bed and below the patient's bladder level, to allow for the free flow of urine.

Procedure for a male patient

The penis is the organ in the male which contains the urethra. The catheter is positioned in the urethra through the tip of the penis.

The end of the penis in the male infant is covered by a loose skin known as the foreskin. The foreskin may subsequently be removed, for religious or medical reasons, by the surgical process of circumcision. A natural moist secretion known as smegma will accumulate under the foreskin of the uncircumcised male, and if care is not regularly and scrupulously carried out, the area surrounding the catheter in an uncircumcised patient could become very sore and foul-smelling.

The preparation for the procedure is as for a female patient.

Hold the penis gently using a soapy flannel, and in the case of an uncircumcised patient push the foreskin back gently. Wash and rinse the exposed area with the flannel and warm water. After drying make sure that the foreskin is brought forward to cover the urethral opening. Whilst doing this the catheter must be held steadily, to avoid all unnecessary movement and consequent discomfort for the patient. The scrotum is washed with a soapy flannel, rinsed and dried gently. The procedure for washing the catheter and removing adhesive is as previously described for the female patient.

It is important to be aware that the male patient can suffer unnecessary pain if the penis is roughly handled. Embarrassment can also be caused by an erection of the penis. If this should happen, allow time for the erection to subside and perhaps wash the thigh first, and then complete washing the penis.

Equipment must be cleared away when the procedure is complete, and the flannel rinsed and hung on the back of the locker. The dirty towel and linen are placed in the linen skip.

INCONTINENCE

Incontinence is an extremely distressing condition which can affect all ages, although the younger age group are often better at concealing it. The elderly may feel that nothing can be done at their age, although for some old people incontinence may be a temporary problem rather than a permanent one. Urinary incontinence is more common than faecal incontinence, and may vary in severity.

CAUSES OF URINARY INCONTINENCE

a) Stress incontinence may be experienced when one laughs, coughs or sneezes. It may also occur during pregnancy.
b) An enlarged prostate gland may cause dribbling incontinence. The prostate gland has a tendency to increase in size with advancing years and may obstruct the flow of urine, leading in turn to an 'overflow' effect.
c) Kidney function deteriorates as we grow older and the capacity of the bladder diminishes. The pelvic floor muscles, especially in the female, may also weaken. All these factors may contribute to incontinence.
d) Shock, stress, fear or anxiety. There are patients who may temporarily suffer incontinence when admitted to hospital.
e) Loss of mobility and frailty in the elderly may make it difficult to get to the toilet.
f) Some drugs increase urinary output.
g) Disorders which cause confusion or unconsciousness.
h) Infection.
i) Constipation is a common cause of urinary incontinence.
j) Injury to or near the urinary tract.

CAUSES OF FAECAL INCONTINENCE

a) See (d), (e), (g) and (h) as in 'Causes of Urinary Incontinence' above.
b) Overflow diarrhoea caused by severe constipation.
c) Drugs, for example sleeping pills and tranquillisers, which affect the mind.
d) Self-medication with laxatives.
e) Loss of regularity pattern.

f) Dietary indiscretion, for example excessive alcohol, milk, fruit or food generally.
g) Incontinence may be used as a means of attracting attention.
h) Disease or injury.

DESIRED OUTCOME

- To establish good communication links with the patient and find out his normal habits.
- The medical and nursing team will discuss problems openly with the patient (if appropriate), and discuss his future management with him.
- Continence will be regained, or dealt with in the best possible way.
- The patient will be able to use normal toilet facilities as far as possible, rather than bedpans or commodes. If bedpans or commodes must be used, the maximum possible privacy will be provided and the patient will be given a callbell.
- Access to toilet will be made as easy as possible.
- Extra aids such as rails or a raised toilet seat will be provided.
- Toilet facilities will be offered at regular intervals, which may be every two hours. A special chart may be in use to record the voiding pattern.
- A careful explanation will be given to those admitted to hospital about the routine and the care that they will receive. This should help allay some of the fears and anxieties.
- Ideally, the elderly will be looked after in their own environment.
- Constipation will be relieved and a regular pattern established.
- The patient may require a high fibre diet.

ACTION TO HELP OVERCOME INCONTINENCE

- Remember that the patient may be labelled incontinent because he cannot make his needs known, for example the blind, those who have suffered from a stroke or those who are heavily sedated.
- Pelvic exercises which strengthen the pelvic muscles may be initiated and taught by a physiotherapist. They should be performed regularly by the patient with encouragement given from the nursing team.
- Ensure that new patients in hospital who are self-caring can find the toilet easily.

- Provide regular toilet facilities if possible near the patient's bed, with maximum privacy.
- Use bedpans only if absolutely necessary and provide the patient with a callbell. Answer calls as quickly as possible.
- Encourage the patient to empty his bladder at regular intervals. Explain that by bending the body forwards, pressure will be exerted against the bladder, helping it to become as completely empty as possible.
- Do not reduce the amount of fluid intake, as this will make the situation worse. What might help is to increase fluids taken in the earlier part of the day, and to have the last drink two to three hours before bedtime. It is estimated that three-quarters of the elderly lose sleep in order to empty the bladder.
- Adapt clothing for easy management. A fuller skirt is easier to manage or easy fitting slacks with elasticated waist without zips. For men, trousers with a longer zip or velcro fastenings will allow easier insertion of a urinal.
- Watch for and report any signs of boredom or depression.
- Sanitary towels may be useful for mild incontinence. Incontinence pads may be used for patients in bed, as well as other protective materials, e.g. plastic sheet and drawsheet.
- Soiled or wet beds must be changed immediately, as must wet or soiled clothing.
- The area of skin that has been soaked in urine may become ulcerated. To avoid this, regular washing must be carried out discreetly and without fuss. At the appropriate time, report quietly to the qualified nurse that the patient has been incontinent. Reassure the patient always that you do not mind carrying out this procedure for him and that other patients need not know. It is not unusual for a patient to whisper, 'Please don't tell my husband/wife/daughter I've had an accident and wet the bed'. There are patients who deny the wet bed, saying, 'I don't know how my bed is wet – I didn't do it, don't blame me'. These comments are all very sad to hear. It is important that the patient understands that all care given by the team is confidential between the patient and the team. Never chastise a patient for being incontinent, no matter how many times bedlinen or day clothes need to be changed. Your attitude, manner and approach must always be gentle, understanding and tolerant.
- The Kylie sheet is a special sheet which can absorb urine without the surface becoming wet. It may be especially useful at night.
- Kanga pants have a special pouch for a pad which absorbs urine but

leaves the gusset dry. The pads are changed when damp or soiled. The pants come in different sizes, need to be a good fit and can be washed in the usual way.

- When incontinence is irreversible, male patients may wear special sheaths which drain into a bag. Some patients may have a catheter in situ, although this is usually a last resort because of the dangers of infection.

In the community a laundry service may be provided for the patient. It collects soiled linen, launders and returns it. A home help may also be provided to help wash personal items.

Deodorants such as Nilodor can be bought from chemists. This is very effective for clothing or commodes.

These are only some of the many aspects of incontinence and some of the appliances which are used to combat the problem. It will not be your responsibility to determine the causes or to decide on the treatment required.

EVALUATION

Care was successful if:
- The patient did not feel nauseated, and vomiting was controlled.
- Adequate privacy was achieved at all times and no undue embarrassment observed.
- Any abnormalities in products of elimination were quickly detected, reported and acted upon.
- After careful instruction and guidance, the patient was able to maintain catheter hygiene.
- Continence of bladder and/or bowel was achieved, or the patient learned to accept the problem and cope physically and mentally with it.

— NOTES —

— NOTES —

Chapter 7

How to Move the Patient and Help Him Maintain a Desirable Posture

TERMINOLOGY

Abdomen – Large body cavity immediately below the chest.

Flaccid – Weak, soft, limp.

Hemiparesis – Slight or incomplete paralysis affecting one side of the body.

Hemiplegia – Paralysis of one side of the body.

Monoplegia – Paralysis of one limb.

Paralysis – Loss of power of muscular contraction. May be partial or complete. Depending on the part of the nervous system damaged, paralysis may be flaccid or spastic. In flaccid paralysis the limbs are floppy and there is muscle wasting.

Paraplegia – Paralysis of the lower part of the body, including the legs.

Patella – Kneecap.

Quadriplegia – Paralysis of all four limbs.

Spastic – Increase in muscle tone and exaggerated reflexes characterised by spasms.

The handling and lifting of patients is a major hazard.

Back injuries account for about two million working days lost in the United Kingdom each year, and in the last twenty years, lifting accidents have almost doubled.

One in six nurses per year suffers from back pain as a result of patient handling.

It is your responsibility to ensure that you never attempt to handle or lift a patient until you have been given practical instruction and have been adequately supervised.

Under the Health and Safety at Work etc. Act 1974, your employing authority has a duty to ensure that you are not exposed to a working practice or risk likely to cause you injury, and that there are adequate staff available both day and night to ensure that patients are moved and lifted in safety. Where requested, additional help should be provided.

Following an injury or episode of back pain you must seek medical advice and should not handle patients until you are symptom-free.

Lifting and moving patients without causing injury to the lifters or to the patient is a skill which cannot be learned in a day or from a book. The purpose of this chapter is to help you recall the basic rules for lifting, and to describe a few basic lifts which you will have learned during your initial instruction period as part of an on-going training programme. Your area may have developed specific policies and guidelines to suit the needs of your patients.

Never attempt to lift or move patients without assistance and supervision, as difficulties and weaknesses in your technique will need to be spotted and corrected. Extra help will be required for heavy patients.

You must never lift, carry or transfer a patient in any way likely to cause injury to him, yourself or others.

NORMAL POSTURE

Ideally one should keep one's back straight when standing and sitting, although chair designs are not always suitable for this, and it may be necessary to look at the design of a chair when selecting one for a patient. In bed a firm base is necessary. Feather beds and sagging mattresses are not suitable for anyone with back problems. Lifting patients in bed is the main cause of back injury amongst nurses. When picking objects off the floor, one should bend one's knees and keep the back straight.

PROBLEMS AND RISKS CENTRAL TO THE CARE ASSISTANT'S ROLE

- A need to lift or move patients.
- A need for patients in discomfort or pain to be moved.
- Patients who are overweight, unconscious or paralysed.
- Patients with attachments who need to be turned or moved regularly.
- Those patients who require handling or lifting may also be confused or disorientated.
- Patients may need to be moved from a bed to a trolley to visit other departments, such as theatre or the X-ray department.
- Patients may need to negotiate stairs.
- Beds may be a difficult size, for example, double beds in the community, or of a fixed height which may be either too low for working at, or else too high and making mobility difficult for the patient.
- Equipment may be unsuitable or cumbersome, or may just get in the way.
- The care assistant may be unfit.

DESIRED OUTCOME

- The patient will move with minimal pain or discomfort.
- The patient is encouraged and helped to be as independent as possible.
- The semi-dependent patient is helped to move with lifting aids, if necessary.
- The dependent patient is lifted safely in such a way as to be safe for both patient and lifters.
- The patient is turned regularly in bed or has his position in the chair moved to avoid prolonged pressure.
- Patients are helped on the stairs if appropriate.
- Opportunities are provided for exercise and activities as an essential part of rehabilitation.
- The care assistant remains fit and free from back pain.

ACTION – RULES FOR LIFTING

All lifting techniques must be demonstrated. The following are only basic guidelines. We have divided these into three sections: Rules for you, the care assistant; How to prepare the patient; How to prepare the lifting area.

YOU – THE CARE ASSISTANT

1) Think before you act. Most back injuries result from situations in which the lifters are not properly prepared.

2) Do not lift patients unnecessarily. Ask yourself whether a lifting aid could be used. If the patient must be moved, check on the most appropriate method for moving him.

3) Do not lift excessive weights.

4) Show patients how to help themselves. For example, patients with a hip injury may be perfectly able to use their arms and the unaffected leg.

5) Decide on how many lifters you need. Do not be afraid to ask for extra help.

6) Get help when necessary, for example when changing draw-sheets.

7) Do not attempt to lift alone – get help.

8) Two lifters should ideally be about the same height.

9) Select a leader – good timing and co-ordination are essential, and one person must give the commands.

10) Wear sensible, low-heeled shoes with laces. Rings, watches, jewellery or pens in top pockets may injure the patient. Name badges may have to be removed. Jewellery other than smooth wedding rings should not be worn. Nails must be short, smooth and clean. Nail varnish must not be worn, as it will chip and be a hazard to delicate skin.

11) Wear clothes which give freedom of movement, that is, not too tight.

12) Explain the procedure carefully to the patient. This will reduce his anxiety and make it easier for him to give you maximum help. Get as close to the patient or object as possible. Many members of staff are reticent about having close body contact with a patient, but explaining to him that this is the safest method should make you feel less inhibited. It may be necessary to kneel on a bed in order to get close to the patient. Make a 'tidy parcel' of your patient, making sure the limbs are fully supported.

13) Position your feet well – place them apart for good balance and to increase stability. Place the leading foot in the direction of the lift.

14) Keep your back straight, head up and tighten your abdominal muscles.

15) Bend your knees to lower the patient.

16) Straighten your knees to lift the patient. Use the strong thigh and hip muscles to straighten your legs and so lift the load. Do *not* use your back as a lever. Smooth application of your body weight and momentum will assist movement.

17) Grasps – use your whole hand and forearm if necessary (Figure 7.1).

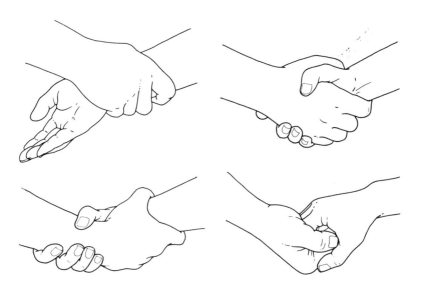

Figure 7.1   *Hand/Arm Holds for Use When Moving a Patient.*

18) Lift and lower the patient gently. Do not jerk, since this can damage you as well as the patient.

19) Use words such as 'grip', 'brace and lift' or count numerically to prepare lifters to take the strain. All lifters must use the same method, and it is vital that everyone lifts at precisely the same time.

20) If you need to turn during a lift, you must move your feet and not twist your body. When lifting a patient from the bed to a chair, pause and check your posture after getting the patient to the edge of the bed and before moving him to the chair.

HOW TO PREPARE THE PATIENT

1) Tell him what you are going to do. This may help prevent tension and apprehensive movements.

2) Find out how much the patient can do to help himself.

3) Assess the patient. Is he fat, thin, heavy, underweight, stiff, flaccid, spastic, blind or deaf? Select the number of lifters required and the most suitable lift or aid to be used.

4) Do not rush. Take your time and ask the patient where he may be tender or sore.

5) In certain circumstances it may be appropriate to ask the patient how he likes to be lifted.

6) Tell the patient what to do. Enlist his help whenever possible.

7) Adjust and prepare the patient's clothing as appropriate.

8) Lift together, so that the patient and you will know when the lift is coming and all energy is used at the same time. This is very important, as you are less likely to hurt yourself or the patient.

9) Watch the patient's face if appropriate – expressions can tell a lot.

HOW TO PREPARE THE LIFTING AREA (BED/CHAIR/TROLLEY)

1) Remove all obstacles and ensure that there is adequate space to lift and lower, keeping your back straight and bending the knees.

2) Height – avoid lifting patients from low positions. Where there are adjustable pumps on the beds for raising and lowering them make full use of various possible heights that these allow.

3) Brakes – are they on firmly? Do not attempt to move the patient if they are faulty. Faulty brakes must be repaired.

4) Foot rests on chairs – are they out of the way when getting the patient in and out of the chair?

5) Space – allow enough space to manoeuvre. Move furniture as necessary.

6) Position – place the chair or commode etc. correctly in relation to the bed, so that minimal turning or carrying is required.

Remember that each patient must be assessed initially by trained staff, concerning how much help is needed and which method is to be used. There must then be constant assessment by trained staff to ensure the patient is being moved and lifted in the best way, as well as encouraging him to do as much as possible for himself.

There is now overwhelming research evidence to suggest that whenever possible you should use the Shoulder (Australian) lift, as this has been shown to be the safest method for your back. When lifting patients up or down the bed, use two or three short lifts rather than one long lift. The total strain on your spine will be less.

Always lift patients. Do not drag them. The strain on the back is higher for the lifter and it is less comfortable for the patient. It also causes friction and therefore the risk of pressure sores, as well as creating added dangers of skin damage.

Do not copy techniques which seem unsafe to you. Always query them.

LIFTING AIDS

These are many and varied and should be used whenever possible and available. They can range from very simple and cheap equipment to more sophisticated expensive apparatus. You will be given instruction on how to use the equipment on your area, but do not be frightened to ask for further guidance if unsure or if you come across a new piece of equipment.

A few items in common use are mentioned here.

Monkey pole or trapeze (see Figure 3.3)
This can be attached to the head of the bed or a wall bracket, or fixed to the ceiling. It is used for patients who can and are allowed to use their arms to pull themselves up or turn over in bed. It may also be used in the toilet or bath. The patient in bed is advised, if possible, to bend the knees and place the flat of the feet on the bed. He should bring his head forward then pull himself up.

Handblocks
These may vary slightly in design (Figure 7.2). If they are not readily available, a few paperback books, in two piles of the same height (say 7 cm), tied with tape or ribbon will do. There should be room to slip the fingers under the tape on top of the books. The idea of the blocks is to add length to the arms when the patient is moving up or down the bed. They are not suitable for all patients, but may be helpful where the mattress is not as firm as it might be.

92

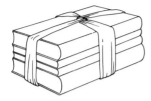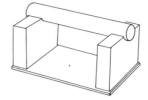

Figure 7.2   *Handblocks.*

The patient needs to be able to sit forward, and if able to do so should bend his knees and push with the flat of the feet. The blocks are held one at each side and slightly behind the level of the patient's buttocks, towards the head of the bed.

Ropeladders
These are attached to the foot of the patient's bed (Figure 7.3). The patient can pull on them to sit up or forward.

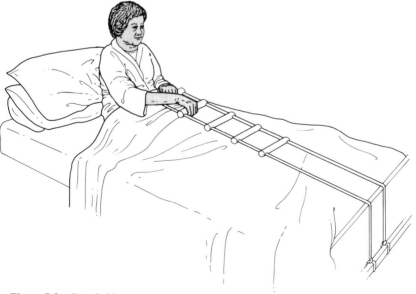

Figure 7.3   *Ropeladders.*

Sliding board

A smooth shiny board to sit and slide on may be useful when a patient is transferred to a chair, bed, bath or car (Figure 7.4). Transfer surfaces need to be of similar height.

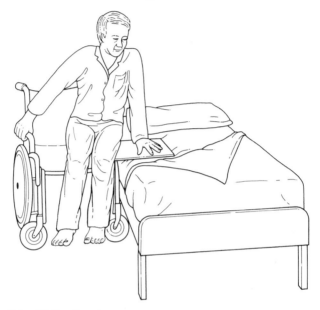

Figure 7.4   *Sliding Board.*

Transfer belts

These can be useful as they alleviate the need to grasp rheumatic joints and sensitive skin (Figure 7.5).

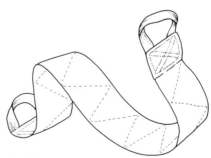

Figure 7.5   *Transfer Belt.*

94

Bathbench and seat
This makes transfer to a bath easier and requires minimal space
(Figure 7.6).

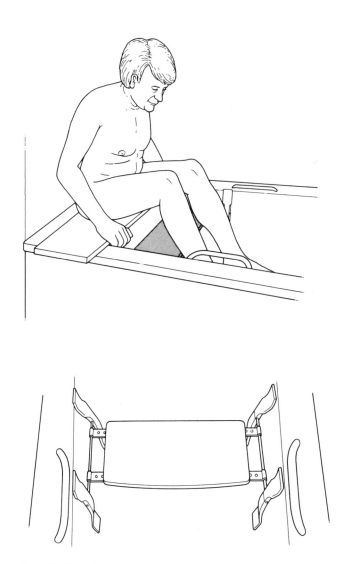

Figure 7.6   *Bathbench Seat.*

Figure 7.7 *Turntable.*

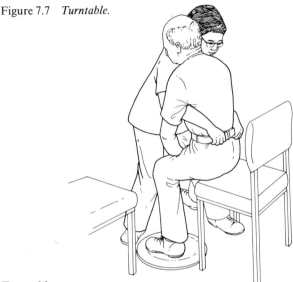

Turntables

These are useful for patients who cannot walk but can assist by taking the weight through their legs (Figure 7.7). They may be used, for example, to move a patient from his wheelchair to the toilet.

Tilting beds

Some beds can be tilted in different directions, operated either manually or electrically (Figure 7.8). They are useful for altering the patient's position or turning him.

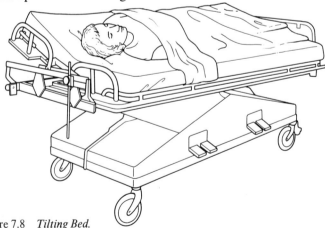

Figure 7.8 *Tilting Bed.*

Hoists

These are many and varied to suit the patient and the environment (Figure 7.9). The design will relate to the amount of space available and the purpose for which they are to be used. Some are electrically operated. There are limitations even to hoists, and most kinds have the maximum permitted weight marked on them. In hospital they are often used for getting patients in and out of the bath, but are equally useful for getting a patient into a chair or car.

Stubbs has shown that two people lifting a patient out of a bath experience high spinal stress. Safety margins are exceeded during this procedure if the patient weighs over 68kg. Stresses will be reduced if a mechanical aid is used.

Hoists need to be serviced regularly. If different types of hoists are used in your area, and if slings are used with them, it is important to check that the correct slings are used for the hoist, as not all slings are interchangeable.

If the patient is obese or confused, care must be taken that any movement on their part does not interfere with the safe operation of the hoist.

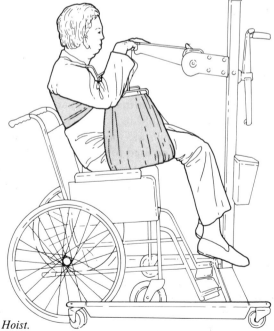

Figure 7.9 *Hoist.*

You must never leave a patient alone in a hoist. Remember too that a hoist will soon become uncomfortable for him, so careful planning of work in advance will prevent undue delay. Not all patients are used to hoists and the first experience can be frightening, so explain carefully what is involved. Never use any hoist without practical demonstration and supervision.

The following general points related to lifting and handling patients must be allied to demonstration and supervision.

INDEPENDENT MOVEMENT

Patients may need instruction on how to manage the following aspects most conveniently.

Rolling in bed

In order to have space to roll on the bed, the patient needs to move to the side of the bed first. He can do this by bending his knees (if able to do so) and putting the soles of his feet on the mattress. He lifts the pelvis up (with help if necessary) moves it sideways and lowers it on to the mattress. He then moves head, shoulders and feet into new position. He turns his head in the direction of the roll. His shoulders are brought forwards, and the upper arm can stretch in direction of roll and pull on the side of the mattress. Legs can be crossed or bent. The patient should then be able to roll over easily and be made comfortable by adjusting pillows, bedlinen and nightclothes. A monkey pole or trapeze can be used for patients who are able to use their arms. It is helpful if the patient can in fact bend one or both knees and use the sole of the feet, because this will avoid friction on vulnerable pressure areas.

Moving up the bed

The patient is instructed, if possible, to sit up and lean his head forward. His hands are positioned slightly behind him using blocks if these are helpful. If not, see if the patient can make a fist with the hands, which should then be placed behind the level of the buttocks. The knees are bent fully and the feet placed flat on the mattress. He moves up the bed in stages, moving the buttocks first.

Getting out of bed
When getting a patient out of bed on to a chair, try to get the chair and bed at equal heights. Position the chair near the bed. Great attention must be paid to ensure that all brakes are applied before the patient starts to move. If the patient is getting into a wheelchair the brakes should first be checked, and footrests swung out of the way. It may be helpful to remove armrests if this is possible.

Moving from a sitting to a standing position
Before a patient attempts to stand, make sure that he is brought forward to the edge of the chair or bed. Position his feet under him and ask him to lean forwards (leading with the head). His hands are placed on the chair arms to push into an upright position. Make sure that walking aids are suitably positioned. Grabbing a walking aid to stand is unsafe unless someone holds the aid. A patient may ask for 'a pull' or for you to hold the aid, but it is better and safer if he can learn to push to get up, so that as he regains independence he will not be pulling aids, furniture etc. on top of himself.

SEMI-LIFTS (FOR PATIENTS NEEDING
MINIMAL ASSISTANCE)

It is vital to emphasise commands for combined effort. You will not normally be asked to carry out semi-lifts until you have become proficient in other aspects of lifting and handling patients. You may then be taught how to carry out the following:

Single shoulder (Australian) lift (Figure 7.10)
The patient must be able to sit up and put his hand on the unaffected side well back, using a block if this is helpful.

If he is able to do so, he bends the knee fully on the unaffected side, with the sole of the foot on the bed. He places his arm and hand on the affected side down the lifter's back.

The lifter stands at the patient's weak side, facing the top of the bed. If the patient is on a low, fixed height bed she puts her knee nearest to the patient on the bed in order to get close to him. She half kneels and inserts her shoulder from behind, under the patient's axilla. Her hand

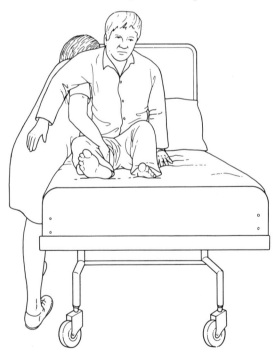

Figure 7.10   *Single Shoulder Lift.*

and forearm are placed either over or under the thigh and holding the upper part of the leg. She lifts the patient in stages.

The patient must know when the lifter is going to lift, so that there can be proper co-ordination.

Sitting to standing using trouser or low waist grip (Figure 7.11)

- Block the patient's feet with the lifter's feet in the position 'ten to and ten past the hour'.
- Block the patient's knees with your own knees – this is easiest on the outside of the patella.
- The patient's arms are placed where safe and most suitable.
- The patient must lean forward before standing.
- The lifter bends at the knees.
- If the patient 'flops' when standing, the lifter should place her hand on the patient's buttocks to hold him in an upright position.

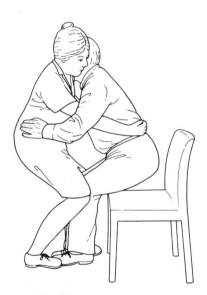

Figure 7.11   *Sitting to Standing.*

A modified form of this lift can be used to move a patient up the bed. If it is possible, the patient's legs are swung over the side of the bed so that he is sitting on the edge. He is moved up the bed in short stages, his legs are then swung back in and he is made comfortable.

Through-arm lift
This lift is useful for helping a patient who has slipped down in his chair or bed. This would usually be done by one lifter but may also be used with two, one taking the legs. This technique may be used to get a patient from the bed to a chair when the shoulder lift cannot be used. It may also be used to get a patient (not an overweight one) out of a bath – although a lifting aid is preferred – or to lift someone from the floor, provided they have not fallen and been injured. You will not be required to assess which lift is to be used under these circumstances.

Lifting up the bed
The lift is easier if the lifter has one leg on the bed, bent at the knee. As well as gripping the patient's arms, the lifter should grip the patient's lower chest with her forearms from behind – this will avoid placing strain on the patient's shoulders and pressure on the chest or bust. The patient bends his knees fully, and where possible, pushes on command with the feet flat on the bed, but only for a short distance at a time.

Helping patients up from the floor
If a patient feels faint and starts to slip off his chair, or appears to be falling, never try to hold him up. You should instead assist him safely and slowly to the floor. You can then get extra help to lift him. Trying to hold the patient up will only injure your back and possibly him as well. Before attempting to help a patient up from the floor it must be confirmed by a qualified person that no injury has occurred. Give him a blanket and a pillow if he is conscious, and reassure him help will be given. Do not rush him. If he is unhurt and only needs minimal assistance, it may be easiest to slowly help him to roll on to the stomach and then push with his hands until he is on all fours. The lifter may help by lifting the patient's pelvis. A chair should have been placed nearby or the patient may crawl to his bed (e.g. in the home). He can then lean on the chair or bed and raise first one leg, so that the sole of the foot is on the ground, and then the other. He can then be helped into standing position and turned slowly to sit down.

COMPLETE LIFTS

Shoulder or Australian lift (Figure 7.12)
Whenever a complete lift is required this lift should always be used if possible, as it causes minimal stress to the lifters and is comfortable for

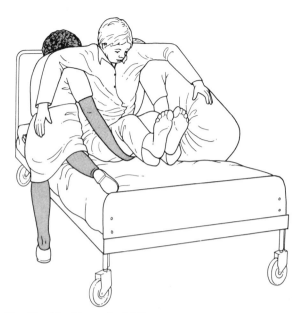

Figure 7.12   *Shoulder (Australian) Lift.*

most patients. There are a few patients for whom it would be unsuitable, such as patients with chest injuries, but it will not be your responsibility to decide which lift to use.

The lift can be used to move patients up or down the bed, into a chair, or to carry the patient a short distance, for example during evacuation in case of fire.

Time must be taken to obtain comfortable and safe hand grips. The main points are:

- The lifters should be of equal height, otherwise the taller lifter will have to bend the knees more.
- When lifting on the bed, push on the mattress using the arm furthest away from the patient to obtain extra leverage.
- Lift in stages, a short distance only at a time.
- If the bed is low, place one knee on the bed (the leg nearest to the patient).

Shoulder lift from bed to chair

The chair is positioned before starting the lift, allowing enough space on each side for the lifters to lower the patient by bending their knees and keeping the back straight. Both lifters must position themselves correctly before lifting and lowering the patient. They should at all times try to ensure that they are carrying the patient as short a distance as possible.

Bed to trolley lift
Three lifters are required for this lift (Figure 7.13). The bed and trolley are placed in the correct position at right angles. The three lifters stand at the inner side of the bed in order to move the minimal distance.

One lifter, usually the leader, supports patient's head and shoulders with one arm and hand, placing the other under his body at about waist level. The second lifter places one hand and arm close to the first lifter's arm at the patient's waist. Her other hand and arm is placed under the patient at the top of his thighs. The third lifter places her arms at the top and bottom of the legs respectively.

The patient is lifted to the edge of the bed first. He is then lifted up and tilted towards the lifters. They move together to the trolley and gently lower the patient on to it. It is usual for the strongest lifter to take the centre position.

A stretcher with wooden poles may be used to transfer the patient, instead of using this lift.

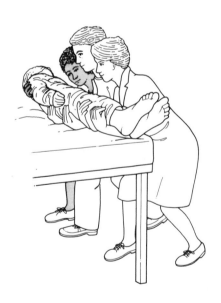

Figure 7.13   *Bed to Trolley Lift.*

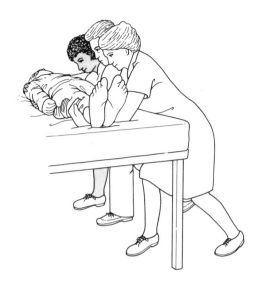

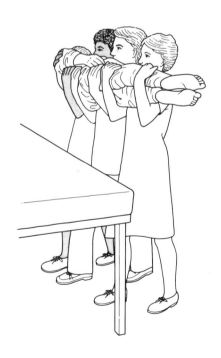

Drawsheet lift

This lift can be performed with a strong drawsheet, a large sheepskin or special lifting sheets, and is used to move a patient up the bed. It is useful for patients who are sore and tender, such as those suffering from rheumatoid disease or other crippling disabilities.

Some lifting sheets have handles, and four or even six lifters can be used. The bed should be in the lowest position for this lift. If a drawsheet is to be used, the ends are rolled up on each side of the patient as close to him as possible. The top of the drawsheet is positioned at the patient's shoulder level. This will give the appearance of a hammock when the patient is lifted. The lifters then grip the corners of the drawsheet firmly. The patient, if able, should be instructed to lift his head. One person should be responsible for supporting the head and for giving the command to lift when all the lifters and the patient are ready.

The lifters start with the knees bent, and on the command to lift they straighten their legs, lean back, thereby pulling the sheet taut and lifting it off the bed. They move the patient only a very short distance at a time, and this way the strain on the lifters' backs will be less. If the patient has a lot of pillows, the lift will be made easier if these are removed prior to the lift and replaced afterwards.

Conventional or orthodox lift

Caution: Research has shown that this is the most dangerous lift. It puts the greatest strain on the spinal column and back muscles, and should only be used if no other method is possible.

If the patient can put his arms round the lifters' shoulders, the total strain will be less.

Rolling and turning a patient (Figure 7.14)

- Prior to rolling, always move the patient towards the lifters.
- Both lifters stand on one side of the bed, face to face with the patient prior to the lift or turn.
- Move the patient's head gently in the direction in which he is going to be turned.
- After the turn is completed, ensure that the patient is in a safe and comfortable position and that the earlobe is flat against the head.

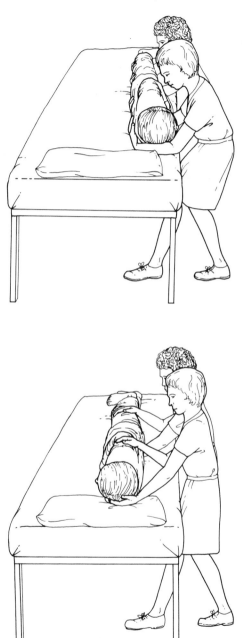

Figure 7.14   *Rolling and Turning a Patient.*

Management and positioning of a patient with a hemiplegia (Figure 7.15)

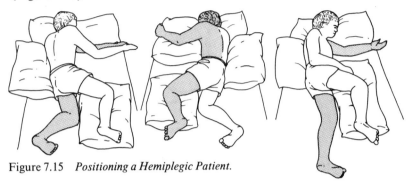

Figure 7.15   *Positioning a Hemiplegic Patient.*

Walking patients (Figure 7.16)

If patients are using walking aids, check regularly that the rubbers have a good tread. Replace any that are worn.

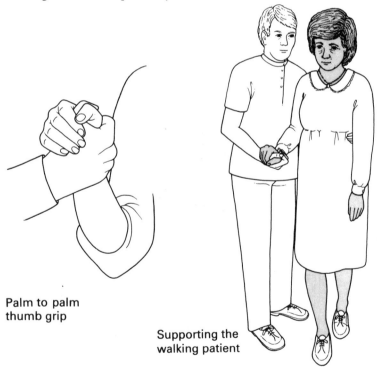

Palm to palm
thumb grip

Supporting the
walking patient

Figure 7.16   *Walking with a Patient.*

108

Helping patients to negotiate stairs

Seek guidance on how best to help the individual patient negotiate stairs. The aim is usually to establish the normal pattern of one leg after the other, but where one leg is injured or lame this method may not be appropriate. When going up stairs the patient will usually put the unaffected foot on the stair first, as bending the knee and using thigh muscles is a strenuous exercise. When descending he will usually put the injured or lame foot down first as he can keep it straight – 'knee locked'. (He might like to be told to remember this as putting the good to heaven and the bad to hell.)

The helper stands between the patient and the foot of the stairs. The patient will usually be able to hold on to the stair rail. To give extra support the helper could place one arm round the patient's waist, or from behind firmly hold the waistband on the skirt or trousers. Take care when using the waistband on trousers not to pull too tightly, as this might injure the patient.

The patient moves up or down one step and you then follow. It may be more comfortable for him to ascend and descend stairs sitting on his buttocks.

EVALUATION

- Was the patient lifted safely and comfortably?
- Did pressure areas remain intact?
- Did you use safe lifting techniques in the way you had been taught?
- Were no back injuries sustained?
- Was the patient helped safely on stairs?
- Was he able to perform exercises or activities as part of rehabilitation?
- Was he accompanied safely to other departments?
- Was he nursed in a comfortable position?

If you think that the method of handling and moving a patient could be improved, discuss this with the nurse in charge and replan care with her as appropriate. It is not your responsibility to decide how a patient should be lifted.

REFERENCES

'Guidance on the Handling of Patients in Hospital and the Community'. RCN
Advisory Panel on Back Pain in Nurses. RCN, 1983.
Stubbs D. A., Hudson M. P., Rivers P. M. and Worrington C. J., *Patient
Handling and Truncal Stresses in Nursing*. Proceedings of Conference held at
Northwick Park Hospital, September 1980.

FURTHER READING

Avoiding Low Back Injury Among Nurses. RCN publication, 1979.
Handling of Patients, Surrey University. RCN publication, or from The Back
Pain Association, 1981.
Handling the Handicapped, 2nd edition, The Chartered Society of Physio-
therapy. Woodhead-Faulkner, 1980.
Wright, B., *Lifting Patients: The Do's and Don'ts*. Nursing Times, **77**, 46, 47
and 48, 1981.
Hollis, M., *Safer Lifting for Patient Care*. Blackwell Scientific Publications,
1981.
Scott, J. M., *You Can Do It* (A Guide to the Care of and Recovery of Stroke
Patients). Ciba Laboratories, 1981.
We All Need To Move, Nottingham University Medical School. Sony video
cassette and booklet, 1982.

— NOTES —

— NOTES —

Chapter 8

Sleep and Rest

NORMAL SLEEP

No one seems to know how much or how little sleep we need.

There are great variations, however. Hospital patients may require extra sleep and rest periods during the day, firstly because of their illness and secondly because of disturbance and a strange environment at night.

PROBLEMS

Bailey's study 'Sleep and the Hospital Patient' (1981) showed that there was an increased need for rest after an operation, but that the increased level of disturbance in hospital made this ideal very difficult to achieve. Patients had insufficient sleep because of noise due to such factors as:

- Nurses walking up and down wards at night.
- Careless use of equipment in kitchen and clinical areas.
- Care and attention being given to other patients.
- Patients snoring.
- Traffic outside the hospital.
- Patients being woken at set times, for example at 6 a.m., regardless of whether it was really necessary.
- No single room for many patients.
- Heavy meals, or hunger, at night.
- Observations carried out at night.
- Upset routines on admission to hospital.
- Change of environment/uncomfortable or strange bed.
- Change of room/need to share/strangers around.
- Arousal state of worry/fear/depression.
- Anxiety/tenseness/restlessness/confusion.
- Squeaky doors/rustling paper.
- Ward layout.
- Temperature – too hot or too cold.

111

Patients may not be able to sleep for several other reasons:

- Already having slept or dozed during the day.
- A strange bed, different bedclothes and possibly also night attire from what they are used to.
- Lights on at night.
- Sleeping next to strangers.
- Physical inactivity.
- Pain or discomfort.
- Fear of the effects of sleeplessness.
- Lack of occupation or activity during the day.
- Boredom.
- Worry.

DESIRED OUTCOME

- The patient does not become unduly tired.
- The patient remains calm and rested.
- The patient is made comfortable.
- The desired temperature is maintained.
- A quiet room is provided.
- Noise is reduced to a minimum.
- Anxiety is allayed.

ACTION

Soon after admission to the ward, the patient should be given a careful explanation by a qualified nurse about his illness and the proposed plan of care. At the same time she will also obtain a 'nursing history' from him in order to further assess and plan the required nursing care. The nurse will also discuss with him his pre-sleeping routines and sleep pattern (or with relatives if appropriate, if the patient is unable to give information). When these details are known, an attempt can be made to enable the patient to continue as near normal a pattern as possible. For example, if he gets up frequently during the night to use the toilet, the nurse may try to give him a bed near a toilet.

VISITORS

Although it will not be your responsibility to make the decision, it may in some circumstances be necessary to restrict the number of visitors and the length of time they can stay, even though some patients may worry excessively if visiting is restricted. The presence of children can be therapeutic, but not over a prolonged period or if they are very noisy. If a patient is ambulant he may be encouraged to accompany his visitors to the dayroom, so that patients on bedrest are not disturbed.

New patients should be introduced (if possible) to patients in adjacent beds. This can help them get to know each other more quickly, and to feel more relaxed about 'sharing facilities', and will perhaps make their stay in hospital more pleasurable.

Some wards now have patients of both sexes. Although many patients will have no objection to this and may even welcome it, remember that others may become more anxious.

REST PERIODS

Patients will usually have a rest period during the day. Try to avoid disturbing the patient when he is asleep or resting, day or night, unless it is necessary to do so as part of essential treatment which must be carried out at a set time. As a member of the caring team you may be able to help to ensure that the patient is given adequate sleep and rest.

If possible the patient should be pleasantly tired at night. Supervised exercise, if allowed, may be appropriate during the day. You may be able to find out the patient's interests and think of ways to relieve his boredom – books, magazines, jigsaw puzzles and games are often available on the ward. The patient may enjoy writing, drawing, painting, knitting or sewing, but will not be sure if any of these are allowed. You may be able to give them the necessary encouragement.

MAKING IT EASIER FOR THE PATIENT TO SLEEP

- Reading may be conducive to sleep.
- The patient may enjoy a warm bath or shower at bedtime.
- Offer a bedtime beverage, for example a warm milky drink.
- Some patients may enjoy a small whisky or brandy if this is allowed but large amounts of alcohol, especially in the early evening, should be avoided. Other people enjoy a small sherry, whisky or brandy added to a hot drink.
- Large indigestible meals should not be offered late at night.
- Ensure that the patient's bed is comfortable with a firm but not too hard mattress and pillows. Place the softest pillow on the top for the patient's head to rest on.

- Help maintain a comfortable environment for the patient by ensuring there are no draughts and that the room is at a comfortable temperature. The patient may require extra blankets at night if he feels the cold easily, or he may require one or two to be removed or folded to the foot of the bed so that he can easily reach them, should he feel chilly in the night.
- All patients must have a callbell for the night and dimmed lighting.
- Ensure that your duty shoes are quiet, and remember that you may have to carry out some tasks on night duty more slowly or more quietly in order to keep noise to a minimum. Avoid rustling paper or being noisy in nearby kitchens or clinical areas.
- If doors squeak, ask the nurse in charge if she can arrange to have the hinges oiled.

Observe patients frequently during the night so that you can report whether they slept and for how long. This is really the responsibility of the qualified nurse, but patients may pretend to be asleep when she goes round as they feel they must not 'bother anyone'. Patients often feel they can relate better with a care assistant who may appear to have more time to talk to them. A patient who could not sleep might tell you in preference to any other member of the caring team. Your observations and comments will therefore be of much value to qualified nurses.

If you sense that patients are worried about something, encourage them to discuss their anxieties with a qualified nurse.

If a patient seems restless, frightened or confused, be sure to report this immediately to the qualified nurse.

Pain or cramp
You must report all complaints of pain or cramp. However, it may be that a patient who wakens up in discomfort will feel better if his position is changed.

Remember: Some people can manage on surprisingly little sleep, so advise patients to try not to worry about the amount they are getting, as this will only increase their insomnia. Some patients may be getting more sleep than they realise, as long periods spent awake in the dark may make them feel that they have been awake all night. If a patient is in a single room he may like to read and should be encouraged to do so, rather than lie awake worrying.

If a patient has had a disturbed night and is asleep in the morning, it is desirable not to waken him at a set time unless he requires essential treatment.

EVALUATION

Care was effective if:
- The patient said he had a restful night and was refreshed.
- The patient was observed, and the appropriate action taken to minimise fatigue and restlessness.

REFERENCE

Bailey, H., 'Sleep and the Hospital Patient'. Research report, Department of Nursing and Community Health Studies, Polytechnic of the South Bank, 1981.

Chapter 9

How to Keep the Patient Clean and Well Groomed

TERMINOLOGY

Candidiasis (or thrush) – A fungal infection usually involving the mucous membrane of the mouth, but which can affect the respiratory tract, vagina, penis, or under the breasts.

Chiropody – Treatment of feet.

Decubitus ulcer – Pressure sore.

Emollient – Softening and soothing application.

Gingivitis – Inflammation of the gums.

Halitosis – Offensive breath odour.

Mucous membrane – Lining of the hollow organs of the body.

Mucus – Sticky fluid secreted by mucous membrane.

Nit – Egg of the louse.

Obese – Overweight.

Oral – Pertaining to the mouth.

Pediculi – Lice.

Stomatitis – Inflammation of the lining of the mouth.

NORMAL CARE

- Washing or cleansing of skin.
- Use of cleansing creams and moisturisers.
- Use of soap and water.
- Bath or shower regularly and in privacy. The frequency will vary according to preference, custom, job, ability or availability of facilities.
- Use of deodorants, talcum powder, aftershave lotion and other cosmetics.

- Wet shaving or use of electric razor.
- Eating and drinking normally to keep the mouth clean, as well as providing nourishment.
- Cleaning of teeth and dentures regularly, and regular dental checks.
- Use of handcream and care of hands and nails.
- Care of feet – regular washing and drying, and cutting toenails correctly to avoid ingrowing toenails.
- Wearing well-fitting socks and shoes.
- Frequent change of socks and underwear.
- Care of hair – brushing, combing, shampooing, styling, cutting, perming and visits to the hairdresser.
- Provision of clean bed linen and clothes.
- Care generally of unbroken skin.

PROBLEMS

- Immobility.
- Lack of privacy.
- Inability to wash, care for hair, teeth, nails or shave.
- Need to keep the body clean and well groomed while incapacitated.
- Inability to eat or drink sufficiently.
- Dry mouth – collection of food debris.
- Special care for dentures.
- Patients who cannot or must not swallow.
- Neglected oral hygiene leading, for example, to stomatitis, sores, cracks, thrush and other infections.
- Inability to reach sinks and washbasins because of immobility.
- The incontinent patient. Clothes and bed linen to be changed and laundered.
- Special care is needed to prevent skin breaking if the patient is chair or bedbound for any length of time. Special care is needed for broken skin.
- The patient is unable to see clearly, or reach and care for feet properly. Problems cutting fingernails and toenails.
- Inadequate chiropody service available in hospital and in the community.
- Lack of hairdressers willing to visit patients. Patient unable to visit salon because of physical handicap.

DESIRED OUTCOME

- The patient is allowed to wash in the bathroom.
- He may bath or shower as desired or be wheeled to the wash area, and independence be encouraged as much as possible.
- A blanket bath in bed or chair bath will be given if necessary.
- Provision of comfort, cleanliness and laundering facilities.
- Regular mouthcare to prevent the complications of neglect.
- Care of mouth, teeth and dentures as appropriate.
- Shave patient if necessary or provide facilities. (This may be wet or with an electric razor depending on the patient's preference.)
- Care for nails as necessary.
- Care of hair.
- Access to hairdresser if desired.
- Help to apply cosmetics if appropriate.
- Regular pressure area care to prevent breakdown of skin.
- Foot care given as appropriate. Use of chiropodist if necessary.

ACTION

All the procedures mentioned in this chapter will be demonstrated to you in your initial training programme. Some areas of work also provide a procedure manual for guidance, and this can be very helpful. It is not intended, however, to take the place of practical training and supervision. The key points are mentioned here.

WASHING AND BATHING

BATHING IN THE BATHROOM/SHOWERS. WASHING IN PRIVACY IN WASH AREAS

If the patient is able to bath himself, ensure that he has privacy but arrange that he does not lock the bathroom or toilet doors if they cannot be opened from the outside. If he were to feel faint it would be very difficult for him to obtain help. It is safer to put an 'engaged' sign on the outside of the door and explain the reason why to the patient. Patients using the bathroom/toilet/shower or wash area on their own must have some means of summoning help, such as a bell. They must be shown where it is and how to operate it.

Close nearby windows. Ensure that he has all his toilet requisites and towels, and check that the water is at a desirable temperature for him. A chair should be provided for him to use when he gets out of the bath. It is much better for the patient if he can wash in privacy in an area which has a mirror and shaving point rather than having to wash by the bedside. It is your responsibility to clean the bath when the patient has finished. He should not be expected to carry out this task while he is in hospital, unless it is part of a planned rehabilitation programme.

BEDBATHING OR CHAIRBATH

Some patients are confined to bed and need to be bathed by the nursing staff, while others are allowed to wash themselves. You may be asked to help. If a patient is very breathless or has suffered from a stroke, it may be easier to wash him while he is sitting in a comfortable chair. A patient who has had a stroke, and who is relearning to wash himself, will be more comfortable sitting in a chair with a table in front of him, with his toilet requirements within reach. You will be guided by the nurse in charge as to how much the patient can be allowed to do for himself. If it is permissible, allow him to do as much as he can.

Explain to him what you propose to do and seek his permission. Tell him that you will help him as necessary. Close nearby windows and screen the bed. Offer him an opportunity to use the bedpan or commode before you start the procedure. The necessary equipment will consist of:

- A linen skip for dirty linen.
- Soap and two flannels – one for the face and neck and one for the body.
- Talcum powder, if used.
- Deodorant and any other requirements for the patient, such as eau de cologne and cosmetics.
- His toothbrush, toothpaste, disposable denture bowl (if required) and mouthwash solution, and receiver for used mouthwash.
- Clean linen, nightwear or day clothes.
- Nail scissors and nail file.
- Comb and brush.
- A washbowl filled with warm water immediately before starting to bath the patient.

MOUTHCARE

Normally the mouth is kept clean by saliva, eating and drinking, and regular cleaning of teeth and dentures. During illness or neglect the mouth may become very dry. If it is not kept clean, food debris collects, the patient loses his appetite and may subsequently develop halitosis and stomatitis. The gums may become inflamed and a fungal infection called candidiasis (thrush), as well as other infections, may occur. It is imperative that the patient is given frequent mouthwashes if unable to eat and drink, and that facilities are provided for cleaning the teeth and dentures regularly as previously described. Toothbrushes must be thoroughly rinsed after use.

Dentures should be removed into a clearly labelled denture bowl before operation and prior to certain investigations, and always if the patient is unconscious. Apart from these occasions, the patient should be encouraged to wear his dentures unless he is used to removing them at night. If the patient can drink freely, this will help keep the mouth clean and fresh.

It is preferable to carry out this procedure prior to washing the patient, so that he does not spill mouthwash solution over clean linen. A mouthwash, toothpaste and toothbrush is given to the patient to care for his teeth in the normal way if this is possible. Assistance may be given if necessary. He is provided with a disposable receiver to spit used mouthwash solution into, and tissues to wipe the mouth afterwards. If the patient is both able and permitted to sit up, you can help him by holding the receiver for the used mouthwash. Mouthcare for an unconscious patient is described later in this chapter.

Care of dentures

The patient who is able to care for his own dentures should be given the necessary equipment to cleanse and rinse them. If he is unable to do this, you must perform the procedure for him, safely and efficiently.

There are different ways of cleaning dentures. They may be cleaned with paste and toothbrush in the normal way, whereas some patients prefer to have them soaked in the solution of their choice, then brushed and rinsed. Soaking of dentures may be carried out overnight or during the bathing procedure. After the dentures are removed from the mouth they must be placed immediately in a denture container clearly labelled with the patient's name. When cleaning dentures, hold them firmly in the palm of your hand.

Hygiene

BATHING A PATIENT IN BED

Strip the top bedclothes and put them on the extension rail at the end
of the bed or on to a chair, leaving the patient covered with a blanket
to stop him getting chilled and to prevent embarrassment. Never
expose a patient unduly. Remove the nightdress or pyjamas and cover
the patient's chest with a towel. The face and front of the neck are
washed first. Ask him whether he likes soap and water on his face and
proceed accordingly. Use firm strokes when washing, and make sure
you wash right up to the hairline, round the eyes and nose, and do not
forget to wash the ears and behind them. Ask him to close his eyes
while you wash them. Even if the patient is unconscious, you must
explain what you are doing. If a patient is unable to speak or is
unconscious, a relative may be able to give details of his dislikes and
normal routine, for example, whether he uses soap on his skin. If
appropriate, encourage the patient to wash his face himself. When the
face is thoroughly washed, rinse off all the soap and dry the skin, still
using firm but gentle strokes. Ask him if his face feels dry. If he is
unable to tell you, feel the skin with your dry hand. The face flannel is
then rinsed and the body flannel used from this stage.

The arms and hands are washed next. Place the towel under the arm
furthest away from you and wash this arm and hand. Observe the nails
for cleanliness and length, and note if they need to be trimmed later.
(If you are asked to wash a patient prior to operation, any nail varnish
and cosmetics should be removed, so that the natural colour can be
observed. If the patient does not have nail varnish remover, acetone
(which is kept on most wards) may be used. When washing the arm,
pay particular attention to washing under the axilla. When the arm
and hand is washed it is rinsed and dried carefully. Deodorant may be
used if the patient wishes, but some types may irritate sensitive skin.
The other arm and hand are then washed in a similar manner. You
must be constantly on the lookout for any unusual marks, scars or
sores, and report them to the nurse in charge at a suitable time after
attending to the patient. The chest and abdomen are washed, rinsed
and dried thoroughly but quickly, so that the patient does not become
unduly chilled. If the patient is obese, wash, rinse and dry the chest
and then cover it before proceeding to wash the abdomen.

Great care must be taken when washing under breasts as they can
become very sore if not properly washed, rinsed and dried. Heavy,
pendulous breasts must be supported. The most comfortable way of
supporting them is with the back of your hand, which also provides a
full view of the skin underneath. Talcum powder needs to be used very

121

sparingly, if at all, and should not be used under large breasts where it tends to clog and cause discomfort. Any sore or red areas must be reported to the nurse in charge.

After washing the front of the patient's body you wash the genitalia, taking great care to wash between all the skin folds and washing always from the front (urethral area) to the back (anal area). When washing male patients special care must be taken while washing the penis (Figures 9.1 and 9.2). If the patient is able, he can be given a soaped flannel and allowed to do this for himself. You can make a 'tent' with the blanket to allow him to carry this out in privacy. If the patient has not been circumcised you will need to gently retract the foreskin. Wash with a soapy flannel, rinse and thoroughly dry the area and then gently replace the foreskin. As we have already mentioned in the discussion of catheter care, it is important that this practice is observed, otherwise the patient may suffer undue discomfort from the build-up of smegma, with the risk of consequent infection.

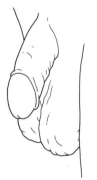
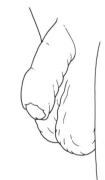

Figure 9.1   *Circumcised Penis.*   Figure 9.2   *Uncircumcised Penis.*

The water must be changed before the patient's legs, back and buttocks are washed. Talcum powder, creams or deodorants will be used according to the patient's preference.

Attention should be given to fingernails and toenails at this stage.

CARE OF THE HANDS AND FEET

Hands and fingernails must be kept clean, and frequent hand washing is essential. Every time the hands are washed they must be thoroughly dried to prevent sores and chafing. Hand cream can then be applied. The patient's fingernails should be kept clean and smooth to prevent scratching the body. You may be asked to help the patient to perform a complete manicure, which may include applying nail varnish. If the fingernails require cutting, take care not to cut the fleshy part of the finger. The nails are cut to the shape of the finger. An emery board or nail file may be used to smooth the fingernails. Nail cuttings must be collected in a suitable container to avoid discomfort for the patient if they should get into the bed.

Feet should be washed daily and the toenails kept clean. After thoroughly drying the feet and toes, a sprinkling of talcum powder may be used if it is the patient's wish. Dry skin may be treated with an oily preparation. Toenails are best cut after a bath, because the hot water will have softened them. They are cut or filed straight across to prevent them from becoming ingrown. If the patient is a diabetic, has circulatory problems or has thick, horny nails which are difficult to cut, do not under any circumstances attempt to cut them, but report this to the nurse in charge who will arrange an appointment with the chiropodist. Socks and shoes must fit well and socks must be changed regularly.

The hair will need to be brushed or combed after the patient's night attire or clothes are replaced. The patient may require help to apply cosmetics.

Dirty or soiled linen is placed straight into the dirty linen skip and the bed is remade with clean linen. The patient is left comfortable, with locker and bell within reach and any other articles required. If the patient wears spectacles, these will need to be cleaned – take care not to touch the lenses before giving them to the patient. He may also be offered a drink after the bath.

HAIRCARE AND SHAVING

HAIRCARE

As mentioned before, the patient may brush and comb his hair after he has washed, or he may be helped to do this. It should be arranged in the style the patient prefers and not the style which you may think is best. Offer him a mirror. After an accident, such as a head injury, the hair may become matted. A little eau de cologne applied to the hair with the hands will make it easier to comb, but it must not be applied to broken skin because it will sting. You may be asked to wash the patient's hair but you must never cut it. If the patient is allowed out of bed, this may be done over a washhand basin. A bed table with a bowl on it may be used for a patient who is bedbound but can sit up. A special 'bedfast rinser' may be used for bedbound patients who cannot sit up. Shampooing the hair can often be a valuable boost to the morale of a sick person. (Figure 9.3)

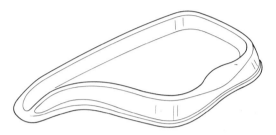

Figure 9.3   *Bedfast Rinser.*

Assemble your equipment after telling the patient what you are going to do. This will consist of:
- Shampoo.
- Washbowl.
- A plastic sheet to protect the bed.
- Towels.
- A bucket on the floor for dirty water.
- A clean brush and comb.
- Jugs of water at the correct temperature.
- A hairdrier (most wards have one).
- Hair rollers, if these are to be used.
- Mirror.

The patient's pillows are removed and the sheet protected with a plastic cover. The bedfast rinser is placed on top of this. The patient rests his head on the rinser. Water drains into a bowl placed on a chair by the side of the bed. This is emptied as necessary. If a bedfast rinser is not available, you can also proceed in the following way.

Method
This should be demonstrated to you as part of your in-service training.
   Get extra help and then pull the mattress down carefully over the end of the bed, leaving a gap at the top just big enough to insert the

washbowl. The plastic sheet is placed over the mattress and the gap and the bowl on top. The patient's shoulders should be protected with an extra towel. Help him up the bed so that the head is supported over the bowl. The hair is then washed with shampoo and rinsed, and this is repeated until the hair is clean (clean hair squeaks). If the patient likes hair conditioner, apply this next. The bowl is emptied into the bucket on the floor as necessary.

It is usual for two people to carry out this procedure so that one can continually support the patient's head. When the hair has been shampooed it is covered by a towel, the bowl and plastic sheet are removed, and the mattress and pillows are repositioned. The hair is dried with the towel or hair drier, and is then combed with the clean comb in whatever way the patient desires. The equipment is then cleared away and all spills wiped up to prevent accidents.

INFESTATION OF THE SCALP BY THE HEAD LOUSE
(PEDICULOSIS CAPITIS)

This is an increasing problem because lice have become resistant to treatment, and it can cause great embarrassment. The risk of infestation from lice is greater where there are crowds of people, as in schools. Although pediculosis capitis is often found in children, it can affect adults too.

Minute white nits (eggs) from the lice are attached to hair, usually on the scalp at the back of the head and behind the ears. When the eggs have hatched they can rapidly transmit to 'clean' scalps and cause intense itching, as they live on human blood. Various commercial preparations can be used to treat this condition. They are normally used as a shampoo, and clear instructions are given on the container. The hair is later combed with a fine tooth comb to remove the nits. Combs and brushes must be disinfected and all members of the family treated diligently in the same manner. The patient must be told that this can happen to anyone and that it is not a sign of being 'dirty'. Treatment must start immediately after the infestation is discovered.

SHAVING THE PATIENT

You may be asked to shave, or help to shave, a patient using an electric razor. This is usually a simple procedure. The patient may wish pre-shave lotion to be used. The protective cover is removed from the razor and you hold the skin taut with one hand, gently shaving in the opposite direction until the growth of the whiskers has been removed from the face and cheeks. The razor must be cleaned after the procedure.

Some patients may prefer a wet shave, and the equipment required for this is as follows:
- A bowl of hot water.
- A towel.
- Soap.
- A shaving brush or plastic sponge squares with which to apply the shaving soap.
- A razor and new blade.
- Tissues.

Method
It is important that you are supervised during your first attempt at this procedure.

The patient is protected with a towel. The face and neck are well lathered with the brush, soap and water. The patient is shaved by pulling the skin taut with one hand and shaving in the opposite direction, taking care not to cut the skin. Excess soap and hair is removed with the tissues. The face is rinsed and dried. Some patients may like after-shave lotion applied, but remember that it might sting on any small cuts. The patient is left comfortable and the equipment cleared. The razor blade must be discarded in the appropriate container to prevent accidents to any members of staff. Some razors are disposable, while others will need to be cleaned ready for re-use. This will probably mean sending the razors to be autoclaved in the central sterile supply department.

MOUTHCARE FOR THE SERIOUSLY ILL OR UNCONSCIOUS PATIENT

These patients require special mouthcare for comfort, cleanliness, moisture and the prevention of infection. You may be shown how to perform this care and asked to do it at regular intervals. The actual frequency will be indicated by qualified nursing staff, as this may vary from area to area. The procedure has remained virtually unchanged for years, but research by Howarth (1977) indicates that the usual mouthcare procedures may have little effect.

It will be the responsibility of qualified staff to indicate what treatment they want you to provide. Remember to wash and dry your hands prior to carrying out any procedure. Cuts or grazes must be protected with a waterproof dressing. After explaining to the patient what you propose to do, screen the bed and protect his clothing and bed linen with a towel. Before carrying out the procedure inspect the mouth and report any abnormalities, such as cracks, swelling, discolouration or thrush to the nurse in charge. Remove the dentures, if present, into the denture bowl.

Two lotions and an emollient which may be helpful are:

- *Sodium bicarbonate 1%* (1 teaspoonful of sodium bicarbonate to 500 millilitres of water). This is an effective cleansing agent which should only be used when necessary, as it is generally unpleasant to taste.
- *Glycerine of thymol or lemon* is made up as a mouthwash solution and is temporarily refreshing, although some patients do not like it.

Note: Both these solutions must be diluted exactly according to instruction. If they are too strong they may burn the patient's mouth.

- *Vaseline* may be soothing on dry and sore lips.

The following equipment may also be used:

- *Toothbrushes* In some areas you may be asked to use small baby toothbrushes. Guidance on their use will be given by the person in charge.
- *Plastic sponge applicators* can be very useful, or else a gauze swab wrapped securely round a finger. Although this method can be very effective, care must be taken as some patients may bite.
- *Mouth trays* may be supplied from central sterile store departments. However, the disposable forceps which will be included tend to be clumsy.

Principles of cleaning the mouth

If forceps are used, mount the swabs supplied carefully onto the forceps, touching only the corners of the swab and ensuring that they are properly secured. If not, there is the risk that they might slip off into the patient's mouth. Swabs, plastic sponges etc., should not be dripping wet with whichever lotion you use, as this could cause the patient to choke.

The mouth should be cleaned methodically using as many swabs as necessary (Figure 9.4). This may be done by starting at the upper right hand side, proceeding to the upper left hand side, followed by the

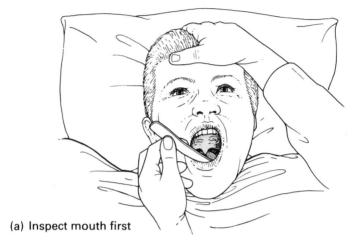

(a) Inspect mouth first

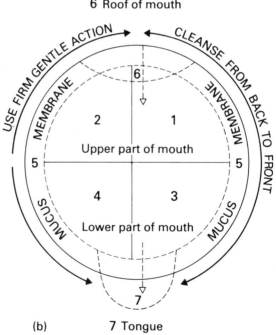

(b)　　　7 Tongue

Figure 9.4　*Cleaning the Mouth Methodically.*

lower right hand and lower left hand sides. The tongue is cleaned last, from back to front, using firm strokes as opposed to a light tickling touch, and taking care not to cause the patient to gag.

Care must be taken to clean inside and outside the gums and both sides of the teeth. If dentures are to be replaced, this is done last. If they are not to be worn they should still be cleaned and left in clean water in a covered, labelled denture bowl. To help stimulate the flow of saliva, a conscious patient may be offered a slice of lemon to suck or small pieces of ice. The patient is then left comfortable. The state of the mouth must be reported to the nurse in charge.

Care of the teeth is essential for the patient to be able to chew properly, and regular dental checks should be encouraged as soon as he is well enough to attend. Patients with badly-fitting dentures may require to have these corrected as soon as possible.

The doctor will prescribe the necessary treatment if oral infection occurs.

PRESSURE AREA CARE

Under normal circumstances, when a person has been sitting or lying for any length of time and becomes uncomfortable, he changes position to a more comfortable one. Certain categories of patients in hospital or at home may not be able to change position automatically, or may not be able to move at all.

Unable to move at all
a) Unconscious patients.
b) The totally paralysed patient.
c) The anaesthetised patient who is unconscious.
d) Patients with spinal injuries.

Able to move with help
a) The semi-conscious patient.
b) The partially paralysed patient.
c) The post-operative patient who has had major surgery.
d) Where plaster of Paris splints have been used to immobilise limbs.

Patients under both these headings are very vulnerable and are commonly known as 'at risk'. One of the risks is the development of pressure sores – prevention is the best treatment. This may be done by regularly (two to four hourly) washing, patting dry and turning the patient to change the body position and make him comfortable.

Pressure sores could develop on any weight-bearing area and over any bony protuberance, for example the whole of the spinal column, the back of the head, the shoulders and shoulder blades, elbows, wrists and knuckles (Figure 9.5).

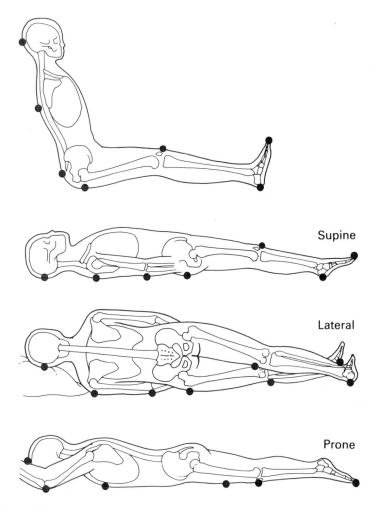

Figure 9.5   *Pressure Areas.*

Many studies have been undertaken on the problem of pressure sores. Probably the most famous one was done by Norton (1975), who devised a scale for measuring patients at risk and when preventative measures should be taken. This is widely used and we describe it here.

PRESSURE SORE RISK RATING SCALE

The patient's condition is assessed and he is given a score, under five different headings. The score is totalled and the lower the total, the higher the risk. A score of fourteen or less indicates patients who are at risk and who require preventative measures to be taken.

Scoring System

Group A, Physical condition
Good–4   Fair–3   Poor–2   Very bad–1

Group B, Mental condition
Alert–4   Apathetic–3   Confused–2   Stuporous–1

Group C, Activity
Ambulant–4   Walk/help–3   Chairbound–2   Bedfast–1

Group D, Mobility
Full–4   Slightly limited–3   Very limited–2   Immobile–1

Group E, Incontinent
Not–4   Occasionally–3   Usually/urine–2   Doubly–1

Pressure, resulting in insufficient blood supply, is one of the main causes of breakdown of the skin. Malnutrition may also cause skin to 'break' due to lack of nourishment. Patients who are incontinent must have bed linen and clothing changed immediately so that they do not lie in a wet bed, which would also increase the risk of pressure sores developing.

Careful lifting techniques prevent damage to the skin, which would otherwise be caused if the patient was dragged. Friction and heat both irritate the skin. This can even be caused by the patient sliding down the bed, exerting what is known as a shearing force.

RECOGNITION OF A PRESSURE SORE

Any sign of redness, blisters, dusky blue/grey areas, deterioration or break in the skin must be reported immediately to the nurse in charge.

Several kinds of nursing aids are available to help prevent the development of a pressure sore.

Sheepskins (pure or synthetic) may be used to relieve pressure on the buttocks. Smaller pads may be applied to the heels and elbows. Regular inspection after applying heel or elbow pads is essential to ensure they have maintained their correct position and that the limb remains comfortable. When sheepskins become soiled, care must be taken to follow the manufacturer's cleaning instructions because some may require specialist cleaning.

Pillows can be used as appropriate, but the care assistant must be guided by the trained staff as to where these are placed. It can be dangerous for the patient if they are wrongly positioned.

Foam rings may be used for the patient to sit on, and are supplied with a special washable cover.

Bed attachments such as:

Monkey poles, ladders or ropes enable the patient to have some independence. He can pull on a ladder or rope to relieve body weight or change position slightly.

Bedcradles take the weight of bedclothes off the patient's limbs, thereby allowing him freedom of movement. A flannelette sheet or lightweight blanket should be placed next to the patient to cover the limbs loosely and to avoid chilling or causing him to get a draught. Bedsocks may also be used.

Ripple mattress. This is a special mattress divided into sections (Figure 9.6). It is made of heavy-gauge polythene and operated by a small electric box which is strapped to the side of the bed. Alternate cells of the mattress are inflated with air at regular intervals of time, creating a constant, unobtrusive ripple and thus relieving pressure. Care must be taken when making the bed not to tuck in the leads from the electric box.

Flotation mattress. This reduces pressure on the patient's body and provides support by conforming to the body's contours.

Water beds. These provide a water cushion between the patient's body and bed frame. They are very expensive but they are also available on hire to hospitals and for home use. The mattress is made of heavy-gauge plastic and contains water which is maintained at body temperature, being electrically controlled. As they are extremely heavy, due to the weight of water in them, there must be a strong, substantial concrete floor for the bed to stand on. It can be difficult to lift and turn patients on this type of mattress. Water cushions which work on the same principle may be used.

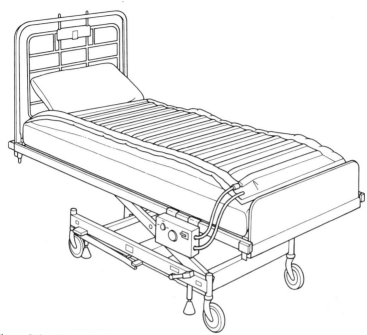

Figure 9.6 *Ripple Bed.*

'Egg box' mattresses or cushions, which allow circulation of air on the patient's skin.

Mecabeds (mesh suspension beds). These are useful aids to relieve pressure with minimal disturbance and maximum comfort to the patient. All pressure points are relieved and the bed provides total skin ventilation. The patient is turned without skin shear risk. The mesh fits most beds without tools and adapters. It is made of polyester and is easy to launder (Figure 9.7, overleaf).

If the patient does develop a red area, every effort must be made to avoid the body weight resting on that particular area until the normal colour returns. Once a pressure sore has developed, you will be instructed if any special treatment is to be carried out, although you will not normally be responsible for this care. You must never yourself make any decisions about the treatment of a pressure sore. If you observe a red area or sore round the edge of orthopaedic plasters, bandages or splints you must report it immediately.

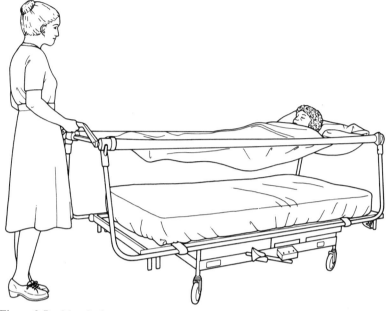

Figure 9.7   *Mecabed.*

EVALUATION

After caring for a patient for a period of time, evaluate the effectiveness of the care you gave and whether it could be improved.

Care was probably effective if:

- The patient looked refreshed and said that he felt comfortable.
- He was given adequate privacy.
- He did not develop pressure sores. Any abnormality was quickly reported.

REFERENCES

Howarth, H., 'A Study of the Mouth Care Procedure Carried out by Nurses for the Very Ill Person'. MSc thesis submitted to the University of Manchester, 1975. (Abstract published in *Nursing Times*, March 10th, 1977.)

Norton, D., McLaren, R. and Exton-Smith, A. N., 'An Investigation of Geriatric Nursing Problems in Hospital'. Churchill Livingstone, 1975.

— NOTES —

— NOTES —

Chapter 10

The Selection of Suitable Clothing

NORMAL CIRCUMSTANCES

- Most people like to be well dressed.
- Clothes are a great morale booster.
- People take pride in being well dressed.
- They like to wear clothes they feel comfortable in, especially those chosen for special occasions.
- Colour and fashion are important to many people.
- People choose clothes to suit their lifestyle.
- The choice of clothing will depend to a certain extent on the weather.
- The type of material is considered when choosing clothes, and thought is given as to whether the material will crease or not.
- Different people and different age groups have likes and dislikes regarding their choice of clothing. Usually they prefer to choose clothes for themselves and to try different styles before deciding.
- We expect to be able to dress and undress in privacy. In public places, such as in a swimming pool, there are separate areas for each sex where people can dress and undress.
- In most cases we take for granted the ability to dress and undress, fasten zips, buttons, belts and other fastenings.
- Most of us like to change clothes frequently.

PROBLEMS FACED BY PATIENTS

- The inability to dress/undress oneself.
- Lack of appropriate clothing.
- Lack of personalised clothing.
- Incontinence causing staining and wet clothes.
- Rheumatoid joints which make dressing difficult.
- Patients may be unable to fasten buttons, zips (especially at the back), belts and other fastenings.

- Lack of privacy for dressing and undressing.
- The patient cannot always have a variety of clothes without them creasing, due to a lack of storage space.
- The temperature may be hot or cold or there may be draughts, and the patient's clothing in hospital may be unsuitable.
- There may be a lack of matching clothing – even matching tops and bottoms of pyjamas when hospital garments have to be worn.
- If hospital clothing has to be worn it may be supplied in small, medium or large rather than recognised sizes, and often the correct size is not available for the patient.
- Laundering facilities may be difficult, especially for personalised clothing. There are not always facilities for laundering clothes on the ward.
- There is often a shortage of hospital clothing. Patients admitted as an emergency may be dependent on this until their own can be brought in.
- Due to illness, the patient may be financially unable to afford the clothes he would like, and if in hospital for a prolonged period is unable to go shopping for clothes.
- There is often a lack of time to dress at leisure.

DESIRED OUTCOME

- The patient is comfortable, has freedom of movement, is happy with the clothing he is asked to wear and with his general appearance.
- The patient is not too hot or too cold.
- The patient's clothing allows him to maintain his self-respect and dignity.
- He is given privacy for dressing and undressing.
- If appropriate, aids are supplied to help the patient dress and undress.
- Colours are chosen which the patient likes and which are also suitable – yellow for a jaundiced patient would be most inappropriate, and could actually make the patient look worse.
- Where possible, the patient is allowed to choose the clothes he likes.
- If the patient is in hospital for a prolonged period he should be able to buy the type of clothing he prefers. A mail order catalogue can be obtained, or organised visits to shops can be arranged for certain patients if their physical condition permits. Some hospitals have mobile shops which visit long-stay areas.

ACTION

- Provide privacy for the patient to dress and undress.
- Include the patient in the selection of his clothes.
- Choose the colours he prefers and an appropriate material and style.
- Encourage the patient to wear colours he looks best in, as this is a great morale booster.
- If possible use the patient's own clothes, which should be clearly labelled with his name. It is always better if patients can wear their own clothes, even if they are incontinent. Some areas now have facilities for laundering the patient's clothing, or relatives may be able to help with this.
- Match items and colours as far as possible.

When a patient has difficulty dressing, you must be capable of offering the required help.

If there is a weakness on one side of the body, say the arm, the sleeve for this arm should be put on first, followed by the head and the other arm. If both arms are weak or stiff it may be easier to put the arms through first, and have a larger opening for the head. Simple aids are available which may help the patient to be independent, for example long shoe horns, gadgets for helping to put on stockings, velcro fastenings, fastenings at the front of a garment rather than at the back. A clothes peg with a loop attached can be clipped to a sleeve, and the loop threaded over the thumb. This stops the sleeve being pulled up when putting on an outer garment. There are also attachments for pulling up zip fasteners.

Many women wear costume jewellery and should be encouraged to do so, although jewellery can pose a security problem when patients bring expensive items to hospital with them. Most hospitals have laid down procedures for the safe-keeping of valuables.

Lightweight shawls are pretty and useful round the patient's shoulders, particularly for the elderly.

Well-fitting shoes are better than slippers, when the patient starts to walk again, as they offer better support.

If the patient gets up to sit in a chair for a short time but does not get dressed, he should wear a dressing gown. Alternatively, a blanket can be spread out over a chair and the patient asked to sit on it. The ends of the blanket are then wrapped round him, protecting his shoulders and the calves of his legs (where patients often get a draught) as well as the front of his body. It is still easy for him to get his hands out to read his paper etc.

Nightdresses and pyjamas are best if they are of an absorbent cotton material, as patients tend to sweat more when they are ill. Nylon can be attractive but is not so absorbent. Bedclothes should be light but warm. Continental quilts (duvets) may be used in some areas.

Aids to comfort which allow the incontinent patient to maintain his dignity are many and varied. You will be advised on the type to be used for the individual patient. These are not the total solution for some patients, and indeed may increase the problem of incontinence.

Commenting on and admiring the patient's appearance is a great morale booster.

Should clothing become too large or too small for the patient while he is in hospital, relatives may be asked to have the necessary adjustments made. If clothes have been provided by the hospital, nursing staff must arrange for the sewing room either to adjust or renew them as necessary.

It is preferable that clothes worn by hospital long-stay patients should be washable rather than require dry-cleaning. Soiled clothing must be separated from clean, and should be rinsed by you and put in a plastic bag for the relatives to take home. Stains such as blood must be soaked before giving to the relatives. If the patient has no relatives you may be asked to wash nightwear on the ward area if facilities are available. Many areas have a tumble drier. A patient's personal clothing and nightwear should not normally be sent to the hospital laundry.

EVALUATION

Care was successful if:

- The patient felt comfortable and attractive and was not too hot or cold.
- The patient was consulted about the choice of clothing and colours.
- He was not asked to wear clothes of a colour or design which he disliked intensely.
- Privacy was given for dressing and undressing.

— NOTES —

— NOTES —

Chapter 11

How to Avoid Dangers in the Environment and Avoid Injuring Others

Infection – Invasion and multiplication of disease-producing micro-organisms in the body tissue.

Resuscitation – Restoration to life of one who appears to have died.

Sterilisation – Process to eliminate contamination by micro-organisms.

It is the duty of all staff to create and maintain a safe environment for patients and colleagues alike. Staff should constantly be vigilant for hazards to patients and all others in the area where they are working, and take appropriate steps to avoid or minimise these. This is especially important in hospital, as the strange environment increases the risk of accidents occurring.

NORMAL CIRCUMSTANCES

- Provision of a safe environment with adequate heating, lighting and ventilation for patients, visitors and staff.
- Non-slip, dry floors.
- Minimal noise levels.
- Security for patients' valuables and belongings.
- Equipment maintained in good working order.
- Equipment used correctly.

PROBLEMS
1) Maintaining a safe environment for admission of patients.
2) Patients who may be disorientated.
3) Area too hot or cold.
4) Inadequate ventilation.
5) Patients' immobility.
6) Visitors to the area.
7) Large numbers of staff working or visiting the area.
8) Wet, slippery floors.
9) Noise in hospital. Use of bells and alarms.
10) Cross-infection.
11) Patients' property to be looked after.
12) Possible need for first aid or resuscitation.
13) Risk of fire, flood or bomb scare (need to evacuate dependent or semi-dependent patients).
14) Equipment old, faulty or not regularly maintained.
15) Misappropriation of equipment.
16) Patients' physical problems, for example the blind, the deaf, and those who have a diminished sense of smell or sensory loss.

DESIRED OUTCOME
1) Sick patients admitted to a safe, uncluttered, neat environment.
2) Safety for patients in bed.
3) Optimum temperature maintained (warmth if necessary, but without burns).
4) Adequate ventilation.
5) Safety when mobilising patients.
6) Safe environment for visitors.
7) Safety for staff working or visiting the area.
8) Wet floors cleaned immediately.
9) Noise kept to a minimum.
10) Prevention of cross-infection. Safe disposal of equipment and linen, and uniform worn as instructed.
11) Safe custody of patients' valuables and belongings.
12) First aid given, or resuscitation if applicable.
13) Regular fire prevention instruction and policy for action to be taken in case of fire, flood or bomb scare.
14) Regular servicing of equipment. Prompt repair of faulty equipment.
15) Equipment is used appropriately.
16) The patient with physical impairment will come to no harm.

ACTION

1) A new patient coming into hospital must be admitted to a safe environment. For example, it would be a grave error to admit a patient who is suicidal to an area where he cannot constantly be observed, or near a window of a ward above ground floor level. A patient suffering from allergies may become very breathless near plants and flowers, so this could be an 'unsafe' area for him. An elderly, confused patient may be unsafe if cotsides are not in position, whereas other patients become more restless with cotsides. All patients will be at risk if brakes on beds, trolleys and chairs are not applied at all times when the equipment is stationary.

2) Patients in bed must have bells, drinks and personal articles within reach. You should try to recognise changes in the mental alertness of any patient, or abnormal movements or restlessness which may indicate that extra precautions need to be taken for his safety. These observations must be reported immediately to trained staff.

3) It may be difficult to regulate the temperature in your area of work, but you can open and close windows, adjust radiators, or vary the amount of clothing and blankets. Not all patients will feel heat or cold to the same extent and some may be pyrexial or suffer from hypothermia. Hot water bottles are rarely allowed because of the dangers of scalding, but if used they must be properly covered, and never applied directly to the patient's skin.

4) Adequate ventilation is essential, although the patient should never be left in a draught and it will be necessary to close windows for certain nursing procedures.

5) Extra precautions may need to be taken when mobilising patients who are unsteady on their feet. For example, if bedside lockers are on wheels without brakes, patients must not lean on them to steady themselves. Rugs may be dangerous if the patient slips, so they are best removed. Non-slip surfaces are best, and highly polished floors must be avoided.

6) Visitors to the ward must also be in a safe environment.

7) It is the responsibility of all staff to take reasonable precautions to maintain a safe working environment for themselves and for their colleagues.

8) Wet floors are hazardous. Notices should be used to warn people about wet surfaces when floors are being cleaned, and spills should be mopped up immediately. Care should be taken where flexes have to be

used. They should not be left where they can be tripped over or pulled from a high surface.

9) It is impossible to eliminate noise in hospital, but every effort should be taken to minimise it as it can be extremely distressing to sick people. Avoid wearing shoes which squeak. Remember not to talk in a loud voice. Patients may be disturbed by noise from the kitchen, and this can be reduced by keeping the door closed. You may be able to think of numerous ways to eliminate noise in your area of work.

10) Everyone should be aware that cross-infection is a real hazard in hospital. This is partly due to the fact that a patient's resistance is lowered when he is ill, and also because there are more disease-producing organisms present. You will need guidance from the trained staff for special precautions to be taken in your area of work, but there are reasonable precautions you can take at all times, such as washing and drying your hands when necessary.

If required you must wear protective clothing. Your uniform must be clean and laundered regularly and never worn outside the hospital or area of work. Never allow dirty linen to come in contact with your uniform.

Safe disposal of dirty linen is essential. You should be familiar with the system used in your area of work. Glass and sharp equipment are disposed of in special containers recommended by the DHSS and great care must be taken, since glass carelessly put in the wrong container may cause serious injury to the porters collecting it. Rubbish for incineration is kept separate from waste paper and kitchen waste.

11) *Patients' valuables and other belongings.* Waiting-list patients are usually advised not to bring valuables and large sums of cash to hospital, although patients who are admitted as emergencies or who live alone may have valuables with them. Procedures for dealing with patients' property vary from hospital to hospital, and you should find out the system for your area. Valuables and property taken to hospital may be listed in a 'property book' after being checked by two members of staff, one of whom may be you. Valuables and large sums of cash should be locked in the hospital safe after being checked, and a receipt issued to the patient. These are returned to the patient on discharge or, alternatively, the patient's relatives may with the patient's consent take them home. When checking jewellery, each item should be described by its colour, e.g. 'yellow metal' rather than 'gold' and the colour of stones rather than the name, such as 'emeralds', as this may at times be inaccurate.

Clothes kept on the ward must be suitably labelled, listed in the clothes book if applicable, and hung neatly in a wardrobe or clothes cupboard. Patients may occasionally have torn clothing, but you must never throw any of the patient's property away, whatever the condition. If you find that clothing is infested, report this immediately. Clothes are removed into a separate bag, usually dusted with a special powder, left for several hours and then washed or dry cleaned as appropriate. You will be guided by the qualified staff as to what is expected of you.

Medication. If the patient brings drugs to the hospital it is usually advised that they are handed to the nurse in charge.

12) As your role is to assist and work under guidance, it is not your responsibility in hospital to carry out first aid or to initiate resuscitation procedures. Your role is to summon help immediately you suspect that something is wrong. Make yourself familiar with the procedure used in your area for summoning help in an emergency. Summon help immediately if a patient does not appear to be breathing, a pulse cannot be felt, the skin is grey or cyanosed, or the pupils begin to dilate. Certain emergency equipment will be kept in a specially designated area. Know what this equipment is and where it is kept.

If a patient's heart suddenly stops beating, this is known as cardiac arrest. The heart can no longer pump the blood carrying oxygen to parts of the body, especially the brain. If the oxygen supply to the brain is not restored within three minutes, permanent brain damage will result. You may be asked to help lay the patient flat if he is sitting up and to remove pillows. If possible, remove the headboard of the bed to make treatment easier. Clear space round the bed for emergency equipment to be used. When skilled help has arrived you can play an important role by talking to and reassuring other patients who have witnessed the incident. Just listening to what they have to say and being with them will be very helpful.

13) You, like everyone else, may feel that fire, flood or even a bomb scare will never occur in your area of work. It is imperative that you are aware of the local arrangements for action to be taken in case of such an emergency. Fire lectures are usually arranged for staff on a regular basis, and you must make yourself fully conversant with the recognised procedure agreed by your employing authority. Be aware of the position of fire exits, be able to identify different kinds of extinguishers, know where they are and how they work. Ensure that

fire exits are never blocked with furniture or other obstacles. Keep fire doors closed but never locked.

14) Report any hazards in your area immediately. Ensure that repairs are carried out promptly, and remove offending items if possible until they have been repaired. If this is not possible, make sure they are clearly labelled to warn people of the danger.

15) Take care to use cotsides and brakes correctly. Do not try to move beds with the brakes applied, as they cannot then be expected to work efficiently. Dispose safely of equipment.

16) Patients may have physical impairments, e.g. the blind or partially sighted. Do not leave obstacles in their way.
Deafness. The patient may not hear the kettle boiling or alarm bells sounding.
Loss of sense of smell. The patient may be unable to smell burning.
Sensory loss. The patient cannot feel heat, cold or pressure, so there is a danger of injury.
There are many other dangers you can probably think of in your area of work. You must be constantly alert and strive to help maintain a safe environment. Remember to observe, record and report hazards and note whether the appropriate action has been taken. If this does not occur, report it again.

EVALUATION

Were you able to:
- Maintain a safe environment for patients, staff and visitors?
- Help to prevent cross-infection?
- Ensure that equipment was safely disposed of in the appropriate manner?
- Ensure that all of a patient's property was returned safely and in good condition at the end of his stay?
- Summon professional help quickly in an emergency situation?
- Ensure that there was no detrimental effect on the patient due to inappropriate safety measures being taken?
- Ensure that faulty equipment was promptly dealt with?

FURTHER READING

First Aid. The authorised manual of the St John Ambulance Association, St Andrew's Ambulance Association and the British Red Cross Society, 1982.

— NOTES —

— NOTES —

Chapter 12

Worship According to One's Faith— Implications for Care

The following brief information is deliberately selective. We cover here only those aspects of different religious practices which are likely to be of relevance to the duties of the care assistant. You will be expected to have a basic understanding of the individual patient's beliefs. You will not be required to initiate or take decisions but simply to assist senior staff in the common endeavour to honour, preserve and respect the patient's wishes.

Patients being cared for at home or in hospital must be allowed to follow their religious beliefs. The particular religion of a patient is usually found out in the first instance by the community sister on her first visit to the patient's home, or else on admission to hospital. This will either be by direct communication with the patient or by the patient's relatives or friends, should the patient be unable to give the information personally.

Not all patients speak English. Some speak very little, and others none at all, and all relevant details must be ascertained as soon as possible to ensure that proper and safe care is given according to the patient's religious beliefs. Patients who do not speak English are likely to suffer a great deal of anxiety and uncertainty when illness or disability occurs, so it is not surprising that patients who cannot fully understand the questions being asked will be even more anxious.

There are many ways in which nursing staff can seek help and understanding. Once the patient's country of origin is identified, there are known people in the community as well as in hospital who are able to act as interpreters, and most health centres have this information. This information is also available within the hospital from senior nurses. Verbal communication is ideal, but if this is not possible there are Red Cross cards and King's Fund cards readily available with comprehensive information in many languages.

145

Most clergy in the community and in hospital can advise on how to contact the particular leader of a religion or following. In hospital they are frequently asked for this kind of help, and will relay the information to senior nursing staff and administrators. Many helpful booklets are also available. There are too many to name them all, but we list a few at the end of this chapter. Local community relations officers are also useful people to contact.

Any bona fide religious ritual must be accepted and honoured if patients are to be allowed to follow their individual lifestyle and particular faith as far as possible. This may mean that specific meals will be required for some patients, and the qualified nursing staff will usually invite the catering officer or dietitian to visit and discuss the individual patient's requirements. Some hospitals arrange for relatives to bring food in for the patient.

Devout followers of any religious faith expect to follow their usual customs in illness as well as in health, and gain much comfort from doing so. There may be special rituals to be performed for the terminally ill and also after death has occurred. The different beliefs will influence the thinking and behaviour of the patient and family, and may ultimately have a bearing on the progress of the illness itself.

ORTHODOX JEWS

Orthodox Jews do not eat pork and have recognised days of fasting. Shellfish is forbidden. Meat and milk foods must be kept apart in cooking and eating. The family may wish to bring meals into hospital for the patient. Before meals it is usual for them to wash their hands and say a brief prayer. Orthodox Jewish women prefer to keep their hair covered, usually with a scarf. Orthodox men prefer to be bearded. Baby boys are circumcised eight days after birth. After death, the leader of the faith may wish to say prayers with the family at the bedside, and may perform the last offices for the patient. Alternatively, a fellow male or female member of the family may carry out this procedure.

MUSLIMS

Confusion may arise when recording names. A Muslim may have several personal, religious and family names. If there is a family name, use it for the records – if not, establish the main personal name and use it. When planning their diet it has to be remembered that pork is strictly forbidden.

Fasting
This occurs during the month of Ramadan, the ninth month of the Mohammedan year. A Muslim starts his fast one and a half hours before sunrise and is allowed to eat and drink only after sunset. Fasting is excused during menstruation and after recent childbirth. Ill patients are usually excused the fast, but are expected to follow the ritual later.

Birth
Some women may refuse to be examined internally before giving birth. As soon as a Muslim child is born, a member of the family recites in the baby's ear a prayer which lasts a minute or two. A male child is circumcised as soon as possible.

Toilet and ablutions
Great importance is attached to cleanliness. Muslims prefer to wash in free-flowing water and cannot accept the idea of sitting in a bath. They need water in toilets since toilet paper is not considered adequate. If a bedpan is used, a container of clean water must accompany it as well as a washbowl.

Prayers
If the patient cannot say his prayers by spreading his prayer mat on the ground, he can offer his ritual prayers while sitting on a chair or on his bed. He may enquire the direction of Mecca to turn his face to while praying. In Britain this is to the south east. Before prayer, the worshipper washes his hands, rinses his mouth, washes his hands up to the elbows and his feet up to the ankles. Women are required to wash the whole body after menstruation.

Family planning
Strictly speaking, an Orthodox Muslim would not approve of contraceptive devices, although in practice individual attitudes vary widely.

Modesty
A Muslim woman may not in general be examined or surrounded by male members of the medical staff and may not agree to be examined or treated by a male. A Muslim woman should be nursed in a female ward. Short gowns such as X-ray and operation gowns are considered immodest, and whenever possible the patient should be allowed to wear one which will cover the body as far as the ankles. Some Arabs

and Pakistani men of the Muslim religion will be reluctant to accept instructions from a female nurse or doctor. If you have any difficulties you should seek advice from qualified nursing staff. You must never force a patient to do anything or accept any care against his will.

Blood transfusions and transplants

In strict Orthodox terms these can only be accepted with reluctance. The decision lies with the individual and the family, and they may wish to consult their religious leader before taking a decision.

Death

It is desirable to avoid a post-mortem if legally possible, as this is not approved. The organs should all be buried inside the body, and nursing staff should ensure that the face of the patient is placed over the right shoulder and facing south east. The body should not be touched by hospital staff. The next of kin will want to arrange for the washing of the body before burial. It is customary amongst Muslims to express their emotions freely when a relative dies, and whenever possible they should be given privacy to do so.

SIKHS

Sikhs have three names – a personal name, a title (Singh for all men and Kaur for all women) and the family name. Usually they prefer to be called by their first name. To avoid confusion in the records it is best to obtain the family name.

Diet

Sikhs do not eat beef. While most will accept other meats, some Sikh women will not eat meat of any kind. It is helpful to explain to patients whether dishes such as 'Irish stew' or 'Scotch broth' contain meat and whether it is beef, pork or lamb.

Fasting

Some Sikhs may wish to fast when there is a full moon, although this is not universal. Men are not allowed to cut their hair and must cover it with a turban. Men and women Sikhs are instructed by the religious leader, or guru, to rise early, to say prayers at sunrise and before going to bed, to abstain from smoking tobacco, taking drugs unless prescribed, or drinking alcohol.

Blood transfusions and transplants

Sikhs have no objection to these.

Birth
Relatives may request that the mother has complete rest for forty days and will be worried if she has to get up for a bath within the first few days, or if she is only admitted for delivery and then sent home.

Ablutions and toilet
As with many other Asian patients, Sikhs prefer to wash in free-flowing water rather than sitting in a bath, and will appreciate having water provided in the same room as the toilet or with a bedpan.

Modesty
Women prefer to be examined by a female doctor, although in case of emergency do not mind being examined by male doctors, providing there is a female member of staff present. To avoid embarrassment, be helpful in providing gowns worn in X-ray or theatre which are long enough to cover the ankle.

Attitudes to medical staff and illness
In general, Sikh patients will accept the authority of the professional, whether male or female.

Death
Sikhs do not like the idea of a post-mortem but will accept it if it is legally unavoidable. According to Sikh belief, all dead bodies are invariably cremated.

It is necessary to repeat that you may wish to seek further guidance on specific instructions and rituals to be observed by other religious sects and denominations from senior nursing staff and hospital chaplains. No patient must be deprived of spiritual guidance, neither should religious practices be forced on those who are not religious. Most hospital chaplains will offer guidance to nursing staff on the best approach to a 'religious' problem, if asked to do so.

FURTHER READING

Dickie, J., *Religious Cultures*, 'A guide to patients' beliefs and customs for Health Service staff.' Lothian Community Relations Council, 12A Forth Street, Edinburgh EH1 3LH, 1978.

Catering for Minority Groups. Health Service Catering Manual, Volume 6. DHSS, Hannibal House, Elephant and Castle, London SE1 6JE. (1627) Dd 8296949 7M 10/81 G 3927.

Chapter 13

Living in Such a Way That There is a Sense of Achievement

Most activities carried out in our daily living are taken for granted. It is not until we are ill or incapacitated that we realise the sense of achievement we get from doing simple things – taking a pride in our appearance, enjoying meals with family and friends, keeping well groomed, shopping, going to work, taking part in recreation, having a walk in the fresh air, or just sitting with our feet up.

PROBLEMS

Problems arise when we are no longer able to pursue previously enjoyed activities, or lack the inclination to do so. Some patients lose interest in life and have no desire to go on. These feelings may be triggered off by the death of someone close to a person's heart. Some elderly patients will feel that since many of their friends and relatives have died they are too old and frail to take up new interests or pursue old ones. An inability to communicate verbally and be understood creates special problems, and patients may prefer to 'withdraw' and isolate themselves. Some people have little if any continuing contact with people, such as elderly widows or widowers, or those who are physically or mentally handicapped. There are many people living on their own at home who are extremely lonely and who may see no one but the community nurse or the occasional tradesman. When the community nurse is no longer needed for nursing reasons it is well known for a lonely patient to complain of another ailment, genuine or otherwise, to maintain a means of contact and communication.

ACTION

Skilled help is needed in order to tackle these problems. You may be able to think of ways in which to occupy the patient and make him feel that he can still do something worthwhile. A bored patient will not be a happy one. With too much time to worry he will become even more depressed.

When you are talking to patients it is easy to converse with those who are cheerful and have plenty to say. Try also to talk to the quiet ones – those who never have visitors or who are deaf, or blind, or have speech problems or get cross easily. There may be games you can play with them, or you may be able to help them to do a jigsaw puzzle or draw. Some excellent tape slide programmes have been made and these may be available from your hospital library or local branch of Age Concern. When you talk to relatives, try if you can to find out what the patient's interests have been in the past.

If possible, try to position the patient's bed or chair by a window rather than a wall, so that he can see what is going on outside. Introduce patients to those with similar interests. If the patient enjoys listening to the radio, select a programme which will suit him – not necessarily one that you would prefer. You may be asked to help take a patient for a short walk round the ward or to take him in a chair to the hospital shop, but never go on your own without permission from a trained nurse.

Setting a patient goals within his capabilities will stimulate and encourage him, although unrealistic goals may make him more depressed than ever.

Occupational therapists are employed in hospital and in the community to assess the individual patient's capacity for daily living. Senior nursing staff discuss the person's needs with these members of the staff, who in turn will help plan the appropriate programme. This could include re-learning such activities as dressing, using make-up, writing or cooking. Help may also be given in accompanying patients on shopping expeditions. Impairment of speech can also be greatly helped by specially trained speech therapists.

Meals on wheels and home help services may be provided. Many areas now have lunch clubs, day centres and day hospitals for the elderly. This also provides some relief for the relatives who may be looking after them. Arrangements can be made in certain areas to take dependent elderly patients into hospital for a few days at regular intervals, specifically to give relatives a rest. Social workers can offer relief in the home situation with such help as laundry services, the provision of ramps, widening doors for wheelchairs, or the installation of a telephone and, if necessary, an extra loud bell for the deaf. The primary health care team will provide continuing support in the community (Figure 1.1).

EVALUATION

Trained staff will constantly evaluate the patient's progress and set new realistic goals when necessary, in an effort to help him to live as full a life as possible. Your own contributions will be valuable – you will be told how you can help the patient and how much he should attempt on his own.

Chapter 14

Helping the Patient to Play or Participate in Various Forms of Recreation

As the working week becomes shorter, people tend to have more leisure time. With labour-saving devices and a great increase in the numbers of cars on the road over recent years, there is more need to take exercise regularly. People's interests vary enormously, and you can learn a great deal from patients about the numerous pastimes they enjoy. These include hobbies such as painting, photography, sports of all kinds, weaving, pottery, knitting, sewing, reading and writing, as well as listening to the radio, watching television, reading newspapers and entertaining friends. Visitors and friends provide stimulation, as do clubs with leisure facilities, public libraries, holidays, and the many and varied educational opportunities, from evening classes to the Open University.

PROBLEMS

- Those who are immobile have to depend on others to help them to get out and about. The blind, deaf and dumb and those with other disabilities need special help to cope with their difficulties and to lead as normal a life as possible.
- The loss of friends and family for whatever reasons, whether bereavement or moving away from the area, can create many problems for the patient.
- A drop in finances after bereavement or retirement may mean that some people can no longer afford to pursue hobbies or pastimes they once enjoyed.
- People may lose interest and feel unwanted after retirement.

- Patients suffering from hemiplegia, paraplegia or quadriplegia need special help to give their day a focus of interest. There is often a lack of ramps and facilities in public places, and for a wide variety of reasons it can be positively dangerous going out in a wheelchair alone. Many people 'talk down' to people in wheelchairs and do not always treat them as adults.
- They may not have easy access to radio and television.

ACTION

- The help of occupational and speech therapists can be enlisted to plan the best possible care for the patient and to set realistic goals.
- Exercise may be permitted within certain limits, although it will not be your responsibility to decide what these limits will be. Sports such as swimming, basketball or archery may be appropriate.
- Special aids may be used for the severely disabled, e.g. the Patient Operated Selector Mechanism (POSSUM) – a special machine which enables patients to type and use various kinds of machinery.
- Library books, radios and television sets can be provided.
- Communication with patients can be actively fostered by all members of the caring team.
- Patients in hospital may be able to paint, make baskets or weave.
- Cooking may be learned from a wheelchair or by using special aids.
- There are special leisure facilities for the disabled, although these vary from area to area. A knowledge of what is available in your area is useful. There are lists of local clubs and societies in public libraries.
- Holidays may be arranged for chronic sick people.
- The number of educational opportunities for patients with prolonged illness has increased greatly over recent years.
- Guidance is available on leisure holidays and sports facilities for disabled people.
- There are now many pre-retirement courses to help prepare people to lead an active and interesting retirement.
- Calendars, clocks, flowers and pictures in hospital wards can create interest.

EVALUATION

- If successful, the patients may well be happier and there will have been something interesting for them to do.
- Hopefully, there will have been no sudden, lasting loss of interest in life.
- Distraction will have been provided from other aches and pains.
- People will be more interesting and will thereby find it easier to keep friends.
- There may well be less incontinence.
- Patients are better orientated in time and space.
- They have the feeling that they can still do something that is worthwhile.
- There is more liaison with friends of all age groups as well as with people of their own age.

Chapter 15

Health Education

Health is described as a state of physical, mental and social wellbeing. These three aspects are all undoubtedly important, and can be achieved in different ways and to different degrees. There are lots of different ideas about what makes people 'healthy' and 'happy'. Normally work, play, exercise and recreation all have an important part in our lives. If we are able to work we are guaranteed some form of financial security to help provide a home with comfort, warmth, ventilation, food and drink. We can afford clothes, and for some the extra luxuries which we so often take for granted. We are able to enjoy a well-balanced diet and to care for our immediate needs, keeping warm, getting enough sleep and rest, keeping ourselves clean and well-groomed, caring for skin, feet, hair and teeth. We are able to avoid dangers in the environment, we have our mobility enabling us to pursue hobbies, enjoy holidays and generally communicate with those around us. We can take advantage of facilities like six-monthly dental checks, family planning, immunisation programmes and various screening facilities.

PROBLEMS

People who work have a sense of identity, and loss of work for any reason may erode their self-confidence. Lack of work, play, exercise or recreation leads to insecurity. This may be due to lack of suitable work or to ill health. Either way, the person loses his independence and increasing worry can lead to ill health, both physical and mental. Lack of finance may stop him following social activities.

- Worry can lead to a person overeating, not eating enough, or not eating the proper type of food.
- He is then at risk from obesity, anorexia or other dietary ailments.
- Poverty of varying degrees leads to ill health.

- Hypothermia, especially in the elderly and very young, may occur. The whole family may suffer and be at risk.
- Patients who are obese, immobile or generally infirm may have painful feet and may also be unable to reach their feet to care for them, or visit a chiropodist for treatment.
- Neglect due to alcohol, drugs and cigarettes can cause general misery and poverty for all the family.
- Special dangers occur for the unborn child whose mother smokes, drinks excessive alcohol, takes drugs and fails to look after herself.
- Problems occur due to dental decay when the dentist has not been visited regularly.
- Patients or parents may be afraid of reported risks, e.g. side effects of drugs or vaccination.

People who are generally at risk do not always follow the doctor's instructions correctly for various reasons.
- They may not have understood the instructions in the first place.
- They may not think that the instructions are important.
- They may not agree with the doctor.
- They may be confused by complicated instructions.
- They forget what the instructions were.

Many do not take the medication as prescribed.
- This may be because they did not understand, or forgot the instructions.
- They forgot to take the medication, or did not think that it was doing them any good.
- They had side effects which they did not think were worth mentioning to the doctor.
- Perhaps they just did not like taking tablets.

There are increased risks due to impaired senses, especially in the very old and the very young, e.g. risks of fire, cold and falls.

DESIRED OUTCOME

- Prevention is better than cure.
- People should be aware of facilities available to detect early signs of ill health.
- People should seek treatment early to prevent complications developing.

DESIRED ACTION

The advice given here would not be initiated by you, but since it reflects directly on the patient's wellbeing you may find the details useful. Qualified nursing staff will actually advise the patient.

- Encourage the principle that prevention is better than cure.
- Make use of the Health Education Council's posters – 'Look after Yourself', 'Stop Smoking', advice to pregnant women, and advice about stopping drinking excess alcohol, eating a well-balanced diet, education about dental care, and so on.
- Patients can be advised about hand washing and skin care.
- They can be told about the value of help from a social worker if there are financial and other problems relating to their illness, home conditions or any other aspect which is worrying them.
- Encourage patients to discuss their worries with the doctor or nurse in charge.
- Encouragement to participate in favourite sports and exercise may be beneficial.
- New hobbies and recreation may be recommended, especially after a prolonged illness.
- If necessary, it may be advisable to recommend a chiropodist. The National Health Service runs a Community Chiropody service, although there is usually a long waiting list. Patients may wish to attend privately and will find the address and telephone number under 'Chiropodists' in the Yellow Pages. When choosing a chiropodist it is wise to choose a fully qualified State Registered Chiropodist. Advice can be offered on foot care and the importance of wearing well-fitting socks and shoes.
- Measures can be taken to prevent hypothermia in the very old and very young.
- It is helpful to ensure that the patient understands any special orders given to him from the doctor prior to discharge. Patients at home should know the importance of taking the correct medication at the correct time and to report any side effects they may suffer to the doctor immediately.
- Watch out for obvious hazards in the home, such as lack of fire guards, loose flexes, loose tiles, broken glass or wet floors.
- Encourage parents of very young children to ask the GP about immunisation programmes.
- Encourage the patient to pursue any recommended routine screening and investigation programmes.

Patients in the community who are responsible for taking their own medication may find that counting tablets for each day ensures that they have taken the correct amount. Marked packaging of medication is now sometimes available for this purpose.

EVALUATION

- Did the patient achieve physical, mental and social wellbeing?
- Was optimum weight maintained?
- Were grants or allowances understood and claimed?
- Did the patient suffer from hypothermia?
- Were parents aware of the risks taken if recommended immunisations were not carried out?
- Were patients given appropriate help to stop excessive drinking of alcohol, eating or smoking?

Although you will not have direct responsibility on any of the issues above, your awareness and attitudes may well have an important influence on decisions that the patient takes.

INDEX